MW01089389

The Easy Anti-Inflammatory Diet for Beginners:

A No-Stress Meal Plan with Easy Recipes to Heal the Immune System

Table of Contents

Introduction

I want to thank you and congratulate you for downloading *The Easy Anti-Inflammatory Diet for Beginners: A No-Stress Meal Plan with Easy Recipes to Heal the Immune System!*

When you set out to find a healthy balance in your life, it is not always an easy path to follow. Getting your body back into a healthy state can be a challenge! And the common diet adopted in the West, especially America, is even more troublesome to your health goals. If you have been eating the "typical" American diet and following societal norms regarding portion control, dietary choices, and lifestyle activities, you are probably starting to recognize some of the negative side effects. The years spent living this life is what leads to your body fighting itself, causing chronic inflammation.

What makes this even harder to diagnosis and deal with is that inflammation in your body is not always a bad thing. In fact, it is something you need to occur to help fight off infections and protect against injuries. It is a vital response that serves your body well. But when it gets out of control, and it has to start "dealing" with the harmful ingredients you are putting into it, your inflammation starts attacking your own body. It changes from being an amazing healing response to an action that can end up killing you.

The purpose of this book is to give you a comprehensive overview of chronic inflammation and how to address it through your diet. Suggestions on where to buy your foods, what to stock in your kitchen, and how to plan out your meals are all included, plus delicious and easy recipes to make your transition into the anti-inflammatory lifestyle that much easier. Finally, the last couple of chapters provide you with talking points on how to explain your choices and additional resources to review for even more details.

As you begin this journey, I want to thank you again for downloading this book. I hope you find it informative and enjoy it!

Chapter 1: Understand Chronic Inflammation

When outside forces attack your body, like a virus or bacteria, your body produces various substances and white blood cells to help protect the body against these foreign invaders. This is the process of inflammation,and it can be very beneficial for the healing process, but then certain diseases make your body think it needs these healers,but there is nothing there for them to protect against. This is when they turn on the body. These diseases are called "autoimmune diseases," such as arthritis. Your immune system, which is normally there to protect your body, ends up damaging yourself in response to these diseases. It does not know that the tissue is actually healthy and begins breaking it down and responding to it like it is abnormal. This is called "chronic inflammation."

There are a few challenges associated with inflammation. Mostly because inflammation is a helpful and necessary process for your body, so detecting it in your body does not mean it is chronic. And not all forms of the disease are related to inflammation. For example, not all arthritis is related to chronic inflammation. The types typically associated with inflammation are gouty arthritis, psoriatic arthritis, and rheumatoid arthritis. Conditions not normally associated with inflammation include muscular pain, lower back problems, fibromyalgia, and osteoarthritis. These painful conditions affect the joints in many instances but are separate from inflammation. So how do you tell the difference?

There are clear symptoms of inflammation. For example, if you have trouble moving your joints, and they appear red and feel warm, it can be a sign of inflammation. Other times your joints may be stiff or painful. Having only one side effect or just a couple is common. In other cases, depending on where in your body inflammation is present, you can feel symptoms like the flu. You can contract a low fever and become chilled. Other times you may feel exhausted or have little energy. Some patients experience a loss of appetite and headaches. It is also to have stiff muscles, not just joints. Again, these can appear as a single side effect or in combination with multiple side effects.

Your immune system triggers inflammation to help protect your body from something that usually comes in from the outside. When your body thinks it is under attack, it releases its front-line warriors, your white blood cells. They head straight for the impacted spot and began responding to whatever the danger is. This rush of blood to a certain spot is what can make it appear red and feel warm. If the white blood cells think your tissue needs protection, some of the chemicals will begin to leak into the tissue. This is what causes the tissue and location to swell.

Sometimes when this happens, it brushes and stimulates your nerves, which is what makes the response feel painful.

When this response is constant, like it is when you suffer from joint inflammation, the lining can swell and then wear down the protective cartilage on the ends of the bone, causing increased pain. This is just one example of the problems with chronic inflammation. At first, it may just be uncomfortable or painful, but if it goes on untreated for too long, it causes even more health problems and illnesses that are not always reversible. It can even lead to death.

When a medical professional suspects that chronic inflammation is a cause for your illnesses, they will conduct a variety of evaluations to determine if it is present or if the illness you are suffering from is considered an inflammatory disease. Some of the evaluation includes:

- Full physical exam watching for joints that appear painful and showing signs of inflammation.
- Medical history to understand the history of inflammation.
- Questions regarding joint stiffness, particularly in the morning.
- Observation of additional symptoms.

- Blood tests.
- X-rays.

Sometimes chronic inflammation impacts your organs which is considered an "autoimmune" disease. The side effects of this inflammation are related to the organ that is impacted. Sometimes this inflammation impacts the heart, causing shortness of breath and retention of fluid. But when your lungs are inflamed, you can also experience a shortness of breath because the tubes transporting air become swollen. In addition, heart inflammation can cause high blood pressure, but so can inflammation in the kidneys. In many instances, pain is a common symptom of chronic inflammation, but not always. This is especially true for organs because of the lack of nerve sensitivity in most organs. When an organ is found to be inflamed, your medical professional will treat inflammation as often as possible.

Treating chronic inflammation includes a variety of options, including surgery, mediation, exercise, rest, and diet. What is best for your illness depends on multiple considerations, such as severity of disease, medical history, general health, medications, age, and disease type. When your doctors work with you to treat inflammation, they are hoping to slow down, control or stop the process of the disease and prevent more pain. In some diseases caused by inflammation, they may also look to help you regain proper bodily function and reduce overall stress on the body.

There are a variety of medications prescribed when your body suffers from chronic inflammation. They are designed to help with swelling, pain, and progression of the disease. Each medication has a different short-term and long-term effect on the body and can be used by itself or in combination with other medications to help you heal. Some of these medications include:

1. NSAID's, or Nonsteroidal Anti-inflammatory Drugs, for example, naproxen, ibuprofen, and aspirin.
2. Corticosteroids, for example, prednisone.
3. Anti-malarials, for example hydroxychloroquine.
4. DMARD's, or Disease-modifying Antirheumatic Drugs, for example, cyclophosphamide, sulfasalazine, and methotrexate.
5. Biologic medications, for example rituximab, tocilizumab, abatacept, golimumab, certolizumab, adalimumab, etanercept, and infliximab.

It is not uncommon to be prescribed these medications for diseases not associated with chronic inflammation. These include inflammatory bowel disease or cancer or to prevent organ rejection after a transplant.

While medications can be necessary depending on your condition, it is important to understand the short-term benefits and long-term dangers of taking the medications alone and combined with other drugs. You also need to work closely and often with your medical team to watch the changes in your conditions. This way they can determine if it is helping or harming your body through the changes in symptoms.

But how does this whole process start? There is typically a combination of influences that fan the flame of inflammation, but one of the largest and easiest to address is diet. Some foods encourage inflammation, while others help your body understand the difference between a real threat and a false alarm. For example, two common ingredients found in the Western, American diet includes high doses of saturated fat and refined sugars. While other diets around the world contain diets with large doses or sugars and fats, they come from different sources, helping these populations fight the negative effects of chronic inflammation. For example, the societies living along the Mediterranean coast eat a lot of polyunsaturated fats and omega-3 fatty acids and a lot of sugars from fresh fruits. These are different than the Western diet and are shown to help the body stay healthy and balanced.

Many researchers and scientists are beginning to understand now that a change to your diet can help you lower the chronic inflammation breaking down your body. In addition to changing the foods you consume, you can also change the amount of sleep you get, the quality of physical exertion, and levels of continued stress to help your body be healthy and less inflamed. While medications may be necessary once you develop an inflammatory disease, you can help the healing process or even prevent the development of diseases, including diseases like Alzheimer's disease or cardiovascular disease, by changing your diet choices.

It is likely that you will not feel the effects of chronic inflammation over when it is just beginning or when it is considered "low- grade." But when it has been attacking your body for a long time, you will begin to notice continued side effects and diseases that could have been prevented. This is why being proactive and supportive is so critical to your well-being. The following tips below are general suggestions provided by researchers and medical professionals to support your body and rid yourself of chronic inflammation:

1. Eat the right herbs and supplements, like fish oils or turmeric, to support your anti-inflammatory efforts.
2. Manage stress through tools like cognitive behavioral therapy and meditation.
3. Schedule enough time to get at least seven hours of quality sleep a night, including a new ritual or habit to help you fall asleep and stay asleep through the evening.
4. Make sure to get plenty of physical activity every day.
5. Stay away from refined foods and "empty" carbs in your everyday diet. Increase the number of vegetables and fruits you eat daily. Other foods to increase include fish, 70% dark chocolate or higher, and cruciferous vegetables like kale.

Additional Sources of Inflammation, Other Than Diet

There is a saying that most illness "begins in the gut." This means, that your gastrointestinal tract, where you absorb the nutrients you consume to fuel your body decides if you are going to be healthy or not. Sometimes you can feel mild side effects of an inflamed and unhappy gut. These symptoms include bloated belly, flatulence, constipation or diarrhea, and pain in the abdomen. Other than addressing what you eat, some things can significantly impact the health of your gut and your body in general. Below are some of the top culprits of inflammation:

- Stress on your emotions. This includes things like panic attacks, sweating at night, and a racing pulse. These side effects of emotional stress or psychological stress indicate that there is inflammation in your body caused by an increase in higher levels of cortisol. When you feel threatened, either emotionally or physically, your body releases a hormone from your adrenal glands named "cortisol." Thisis nicknamed your "fight or flight" response. When it is released, your blood vessels dilate to prepare for an attack. This is great when you are about to take a punch or need to run away from a charging bull, but when you as dilated daily due to a bad relationship or work environment, your body begins to think this "threatened" state is normal. Your adrenal glands and immune system are working overtime and lead to chronic inflammation in your body.
- Stress on your body. Like the emotional stress, your body responds to physical stress as well. This does not mean you need to stay sedentary,so you do not exert energy. What this means is that your body will panic when there is physical danger, like when your blood sugar drops too low from not eating enough or the right nutrients. This

can cause your body to develop an imbalance in your GI tract. You can also experience skin issues, like hives. If it is severe enough, your body will start shutting down completely. This is the body's way of protecting itself and making sure nutrients get to the most vital organs for survival. When you bring nutrients back in and restore fuel to the body, it should return to normal. But when you make it a habit of skipping meals or allowing your body to experience physical stress often, it is possible to develop an imbalanced immune system habit that is hard to correct.

- Digestion problems. Almost all chronic inflammation stems from the gut, meaning your digestion is probably your first identifier that something is wrong. This is why it makes sense that with most illnesses, your elimination changes and is used as a tool for understanding exactly what is wrong. The turmoil in your gut may be all that you need to address in order to "solve" the other problems you are experiencing. The anti-inflammatory diet is especially beneficial in this situation because it encourages an increase in your fatty acid and probiotic intake. In addition, most anti-inflammatory diets also encourage an increase in physical activity to help "jumpstart" the GI tract to work properly once more.

- The levels of your blood sugar and glucose. It is a common understanding within the medical community today that the glucose levels and insulin levels in the body are connected to chronic inflammation. This is why most patients that have developed type-2 diabetes are also chronically inflamed, and potentially have other health issues occurring, like obesity. Stabilizing your blood sugar and insulin levels are critical to helping your body stay healthy.

- Allergies to foods. Some people are sensitive or allergic to certain foods. Some foods are more harmful to people than others, like dairy and wheat. Dairy's casein and wheat's gluten can cause significant digestion issues as well as other inflammatory side effects throughout the body. There are two options for individuals that suffer from food allergies or sensitivities; cut those troublesome foods out altogether or balance the gut with probiotics,so it has enough "good" bacteria to neutralize the triggers.

- Hormonal imbalance. When your body's natural hormones are out of balance, the body can become inflamed. The most common hormonal imbalances occur with certain levels of testosterone, progesterone, and estrogen. Women who are experiencing menopause often struggle with hormonal imbalances, which is why many women experience acne or gain unwanted weight during this time. It is also common for menopausal women to develop osteoporosis at this time, as well.

- Exposure to synthetic materials. Again, like food allergies, some people may be allergic or sensitive to man-made materials, like plastic or latex. Your body may react to these synthetics without you realizing, especially when exposed to them consistently over a period of time, or it may be obvious that you are suffering from inflammation because of the artificial item, like a type of adhesive or gloves. Sometimes the response is on your skin while other times it manifests internally as shortness of breath or lightheadedness.

- Chemical exposure. This is not just being exposed to harsh chemicals in a science lab. Cleaning products and scented candles can cause chronic inflammation. It is especially harmful to you if you can absorb the chemical through the skin, like through cosmetics or lotions. Spraying a chemical air freshener can cause irritants to get into your lungs, causing lung inflammation. The foundation you put on your face or the soap you use to wash your body may contain harsh chemicals that cause skin inflammation. These chemicals can exist in the water and air, at your work or in your home. It is important to recognize the inflammatory symptoms that these can cause,so you know what to avoid in the future.

- Improper nutritional intake. Foods that are rich and full of additives taste great and tell your body that they are good, but in reality, they are taxing your internal operating system more than it needs. And when you do this over and over, multiple times a day for years on end, your body begins to wear down faster from the chronic inflammation you are fanning. To be able to digest a meal high in "unhealthy" fats and refined sugars, your body has to work harder than with healthy alternatives. This negatively impacts your gut and metabolism and creates a breeding ground for inflammation.
- Foods are known to trigger inflammation. There are definitely foods that are bad for you that you should cut out, but then there are some foods that are not really "bad" for you, but they can exacerbate inflammation. They can cause and prompt inflammation. For example, the linoleic acid found in various oils can cause your body to respond with inflammation. These oils are typically refined seed oils like peanut, soy, corn, sunflower, and safflower. In other body types, a diet with a large number of carbohydrates may encourage inflammation. It is important to observe how your body responds and feels after eating certain foods to make sure you avoid foods that inflame your system.

Just remember, not all forms of inflammation are bad for you! What you want to target is chronic inflammation that is hurting your body, not the kind fighting off a cold or protecting you from injury. This means knowing your body and paying attention to its signals.

Chapter 2: Empowered Eating for Healthy Eating

Most people experience some degree of mindless eating. Thisis often connected to eating that occurs when you are depressed, bored, anxious, lonely, frustrated, angry, or stressed. It is also sometimes called "emotional eating," and can cause devastating consequences to your health and self-esteem. For over ¾ of those that experience overeating, it is tied to your emotional response to something. And unfortunately, some foods are like a drug to your body. They give you a short-term boost to your emotional state, so you keep going back to it time and time again when you need to cope with something.

This response is connected to your cravings for certain foods for this reason. You may beat yourself for always giving in to your cravings for foods that you know are unhealthy, like a candy bar or a portion of salty snack food, but in reality, your body is sending strong, survival-like messages that can push you to grab that bag or carton. Once you begin to recognize these messages for what they are and can observe these cravings and habits, you can begin the transformative process of empowered eating.

When you give in to a food craving, it does not mean you have poor willpower or that you are not strong enough to fight the urges. It is important that you begin the process of empowered eating by quieting this negative voice telling you that you "failed" each time you eat something you know you should not. Instead, be compassionate with yourself. Try to act like an outsider and observe your responses and cravings instead of judging them. Sometimes writing these observations down in a journal is helpful to your non-judgmental, observational process. When you begin this process and change your perspective, the relationship you have with food turns from negative to positive. It begins to remove the drama about food that you do not need in your life.

Part of the change to your perspective is understanding that the cravings you are experiencing at different times are actually a message from your body that needs to be decoded. Sometimes the craving is about a nutrient that you need while other times it is about an emotional response that you need to address. Through your life, these messages can be overwhelming, and you also may not have always known how to trust what your body is telling you. A lot of people learn how to ignore their internal messaging system or find responses to the messages that seem to satisfy the needs, but in reality, only reinforce negative and harmful habits. Sometimes this happens out of necessity because you cannot get the nutrients it needs so you fill your body with what you can, while other times you are trying to follow a certain fad diet and therefore push aside cravings because of the "rules" of your eating plan. This latter example has good intentions and can be good for your body, but can also be harmful if you are not following a healthy plan.

Empowered eating is all about listening to these messages and decoding them properly. This way you can adapt to the ever-changing needs of your body by providing it with the responses it needs to be healthy and happy. For example, when you are bored, you recognize that state and choose to do something different, rather than reach for the bag of chips. Maybe you are craving a sweet cookie, and you recognize that you need more water or fruit. Each moment you receive a message from your body that relates to food is an opportunity for you to observe what it is your body is really saying too. You are capable of gaining empowered eating and leave emotional or mindless eating in the past. It just takes self-compassion, non-judgment, and observation to figure it all out.

The struggle with your health and relationship with food is not something you have to suffer with alone. Even if you know all there is to know about nutrition and food. You can still struggle with making empowered choices throughout your day. It is amazing how many people spend hours trying to learn what and how to eat healthy, including spending a lot of time lamenting over a negative body image and comparing their image with others that they view as "ideal." In addition, many people spend large amounts of time looking for "hacks" or "quick fixes" to their weight and body image so they can achieve their "preferred" appearance fast. What is so unfortunate about this is that health is not always the primary reason for changing your lifestyle or diet, it is appearance. This makes the process of learning about food and exercise skewed. Even if you have the healthiest lifestyle in the world, you can still suffer from a negative body image, and vice versa. Empowered eating is not about achieving your "perfect" body image fast; it is about finding your body as it is and in a healthy way.

Having a negative view of your body can quietly control how you live your life. If you struggle with a negative self-perception of your physical image, you can find yourself obsessing over the foods you eat in order to keep your weight "under control," or end up binging on foods after a period of severe restrictions. This is usually after you decide, "Screw it!" and reach for the foods you know you should avoid. You might also spend extended amounts of time reviewing recipes and exercise plans to make you feel more in control of your appearance. These are all reactions to the idea that you are not ok as you are and that your body is not enough.

And another trap that exists, especially fueled by societal messaging, is that when you finally reach this ideal body image, you will be happy. In addition, popular media promotes that self-love is reserved for those that have a body that looks a certain way. This mentality seems to suck the spirit, emotions and mental strength from most people. This is why embracing a new way of relating to food,and your body is important but hard. It is worth embracing a new pattern of eating and accepting your body as it changes to a healthy existence.

Some of the steps you need to follow to help change your relationship to your eating habits and embrace an empowered way of eating include:

- Do not use the scale as a way to affirm or reveal how you are doing.
- Do not jump from one fad detox or diet to the next.
- Stop comparing yourself to others, especially media images of other people.
- Avoid rigid rules regarding food that you are not willing to re-examine.
- Quit thinking about your weight all the time.
- Avoid eating habits that cause you pain and discomfort.

- Release the extra weight you are holding on to because of stress. This means you need to find ways to handle stress other than eating!

Challenge the misconception that you are the exception to the rule and that your happiness and self-love are connected to the number on a scale and your image of the "perfect" body. You can shift the perception of eating to one of empowerment and healthy support. Do not feel stuck in a rut or keep trying the same thing you always do. This stagnant situation is a result of you trying the same types of things over and over again. Take time to develop your idea of the "ideal" body beyond how it looks on the outside or what a scale says. Shift your focus to being healthy and listening to the messages of your body instead.

A Collection of Professionals on How to Eat with Empowerment

Several professionals believe in empowered eating for your health. Below is some of who speak directly on what empowered eating means to them:

- Michelle May: "It is an intentional shift from fear-based, restrictive decision-making to fearless, mindful decision-making. It is an inside-out approach that guides us to balance eating for nourishment with eating for enjoyment to fuel the vibrant life we crave."

- Cathy Wang: "To me, eating empowerment is the process of learning to meet one's needs for physical and emotional nourishment. It's gaining the strength and freedom to eat food for health, for pleasure, and greater connection with yourself and others around you. Eating empowerment is being compassionate to yourself, honoring your true needs, and setting boundaries to protect what's important.

- Joe Bernstein: "Feeling free to eat what I want, when I want. Knowing that pleasure, cravings, and appetite are all my friends and connected to deep intuition and deep needs. Having the mindfulness to eat in a way that I feel good about and the compassion to love myself through the moments or periods where my food and eating choices don't align with my life vision or values. Learning and growing through everybody or food-based obstacle or challenge. Having a relationship with food and body that enables me to thrive, not just survive."

- Julie Duffy Dillon: "Eating empowerment means choosing ways to take care of our body including food and movement that comes from a place of self-compassion. The food choices themselves are a moot point."
- Cathleen Meredith: "Healing the disconnection with food, the abuse of it, and blind eating: eating without thought or consideration of what it's doing to your body.

What is evident in all these testaments about empowered eating is that you need to work on your relationship to food and the freedom you create for yourself to eat what you need to eat according to your body signals. Before you can change your relationship and self-talk, you need to identify or recognize it. Once you learn about how you respond to situations and challenges, you can begin creating new habits and responses that align with your goal of health and happiness. The beautiful thing about this perception reframing is that you are not going to be "better as soon as..." You are great just the way you are today! The moment you read these words, observe how you just talked to yourself, where you like, "Heck yes! I am great! And going to be even greater!" or were you like, "Ha! Yeah, ok. Sure I am. But I will be once I get this thing going."Wherever you are at, that is ok. But your observation will give you a good jumping off point for how you can start reframing your attitude towards food and the way you talk to yourself.

You are great right now because you are looking at not just finding a quick fix or a patch for the challenges you are facing, whether that is your weight or your health. You are exploring how you can take charge of your health and well-being through health and empowered means, and that investigation is awesome! You are doing something that is great for yourself and your body, and that alone makes you pretty great! Or maybe you are here to learn for someone else, and that also makes you great. See where this is going? Whatever has brought you here now makes you a great person, and wonderful just as you are. And as you focus on your health and positive lifestyle choices, you continue to be amazing. It is a perpetual path or awesomeness that you are walking, and you should not forget that as you keep moving forward.

Food Choices That Can Empower You for a Healthy Lifestyle

The following tips identify several fundamentals choices you can make to support a healthier lifestyle. They are not "rules" but rather guides for helping you make empowered choices every day in relationship to food. To begin, it is important to understand the key to healthy living is a balance. If you eat or drink too much, you overwhelm your body,but if you do not eat enough, you deny it what it needs to function properly. This means you need balance in the number of calories you take in and the foods you choose to fuel it. Apply this understanding to the following foundational concepts:

1. Whole grain carbs are your base. Potatoes with skin, whole grain bread and cereals, and whole grain pasta are all excellent choices to provide about 1/3 of the food you can eat. These help you fill up and stay full while offering a good dose of fiber. These foods alone are not the "fattening" foods you may have thought they were; it is usually the things you add to them. These carbs are some of the best to found your diet.

2. Fresh fruit and vegetables are important. Cut up a banana over whole grain oatmeal in the morning; eat an apple on

26

the way into work, etc. You want to get about five servings in of fruits and veggies every day. Take time to identify times and ways you can integrate these into your daily living. It might surprise you how easy it is to make sure you get what you need without feeling you have to "sacrifice" for it.

3. Eat oily fish a couple of times every week. These types of seafood are great sources of minerals and vitamins, including omega-3 fatty acids, which help support your heart and combat chronic inflammation. Consider the following fish for a few of your weekly dishes:
   a. Pilchards
   b. Sardines
   c. Herring
   d. Trout
   e. Mackerel
   f. Salmon

4. Minimize the amount of sugar and fat you consume. Fat is important to eat, but it needs to be the "right" fats. Saturated fat raises your blood's cholesterol and your risk of cardiac disease. Thisis found in a lot of the tasty, but "dangerous" foods, including; sausage, biscuits, cake, hard cheeses, pies, butter, and cream. Instead, look for healthier fat sources, like avocado, oily fish, and vegetable oil. Choose grilled over fried, lean over fatty, and oil over

butter, if you can. Sugar, the other sneaky culprit in a lot of food, raises your risk of a variety of problems, like tooth decay and obesity. You can guess that sugar is found in drinks like soda and alcoholic cocktails and foods like cakes and brownies, but it can also sneak into places you would least expect, like salad dressings and slices of bread. Most packaged or pre-made foods are high in sugar, so make sure you read the labels carefully.

5. Also, consider cutting down on the salt intake on a daily basis. Salt is known to raise blood pressure and negatively impact your heart health. It can also make you feel bloated and retain fluids. You may not reach for the table salt shaker often, but that does not mean you are not getting a lot of salt in your diet every day. The majority of the salt you eat each day is already added to your food for you, like in cereal, sauce, bread, and soups.

6. Do not skip meals and eat when you know you are hungry. This means you need to pay attention to the messages from your body. Are you really hungry or are you bored/upset/depressed/thirsty? Try drinking a cup of water and waiting a few minutes to decide if you are actually hungry. Or get up and go for a five-minute walk before grabbing a snack in between meals, but do not deny your body the nutrients it is asking for and needs! Skipping a meal, especially breakfast sets you up for

painful hunger messages and cravings that can be hard to deal with. Keep your body well fueled,and you will be in a much happier and healthier state of being!

Chapter 3: Inflammatory Action Plans

When you are fighting inflammation, you know it is a real fight. There is so much going on in your body and mind all the time that it can be overwhelming and often exhausting. There is a reason for fatigue as a symptom of inflammation, after all! Throughout this book and your research, you will encounter a variety of tips and techniques for helping you embrace the anti-inflammatory lifestyle and live a healthier life, but even that can be overwhelming. One of the most important tips you can ever receive when in this fight is to create your own action plan.

This means you need to do more than just say out loud that you are going to start focusing on your health and reducing the impact of chronic inflammation in your life. It is looking at how you are actually going to implement it in your life. This includes developing a statement that is specific and actionable. One example is addressing your water consumption. You cannot just say you are going to drink more water every day. You need to determine how much and how you will drink more water every day. Use this simple water example to help develop an actionable and realistic plan using the steps below:

1. Identify what you are currently doing, and be honest! For the water example, how much water do you currently

drink? Do not try to be "good" during your observational period, be real. How much do you average throughout a few days? Being honest and really helps you create a baseline that you will build on. If you cheat and try to do more than you normally do during this time, you will only set yourself up for failure. Instead, do what you normally do and start from there.

2. What do you want to be doing that you can actually accomplish? This is stating the exact thing you want to improve. You do not say here, "drink more water." You say something like, "Increase the amount of water I drink each day from five cups to eight." Or "Drink at least nine cups of water per day." Be specific and realistic when defining your goal.

3. How do you plan on achieving this goal? Are you going to set an alarm to remind you to drink a cup or two of water? Or do you want a new water bottle that you can fill with your daily amount of water that you can sip on throughout the day, making sure it is empty by the time you go to bed? You need to specify how you plan on keeping track of how you are achieving your goal and what you are going to use to help you get there. This may change as you start working towards your goal, but the idea is being specific about what you want to try. For example, if you find a big water bottle is unrealistic for

you to carry around all day, maybe you find a smaller water bottle that you know you need to fill up three times throughout the day, so you set an alarm to remind you to finish and refill during the day. This means you change the "how" portion of your plan, but not the goal.

Keep your eye on the small, achievable actions that you can take to reach your larger health goals. Apply this formula to the changes you plan to make while following the anti-inflammatory diet. Think about how you would approach your fruit and vegetable consumption or the inclusion of fish per week. Address how you plan on cutting out sugars and saturated fats or handling special occasions and the temptations that are sure to present themselves. Do not overwhelm yourself with a million different action plans, but rather select a couple to focus on and keep adding on to your healthy focus as you develop new anti-inflammatory habits.

Remember, this is your life and your relationship with food. Each person is different,and your body may respond to foods differently than someone else. This means that your plan may not look like another's, and that is ok! Select a change that you want to make, and work your way into your own personalized plan. Once you find a change and "how" that works for your life and needs, move on to the next. Below are some different changes you can choose from that will help you with adopting the anti-inflammatory diet. Some are "Do's" while others are "Do nots." Select what you want to start with and then work through the three steps outlined above before coming up with the next one you want to work on.

Suggested General Places to Focus On:

- Replace foods in your daily diet with foods known to help reduce inflammation.
- Increase the amount of organic food you purchase from the store each week.
- Add more fiber to your daily meals and snacks.
- Add a probiotic supplement to your morning routine.
- Change your cooking oil to safflower or extra virgin olive oil.
- Do not drink more than five cups of coffee a day.
- Minimize the amount of added sugar you consume daily.
- Do not eat fast food.
- Cut down on the "junk" food you eat each day or week.
- Clean out your pantry and fridge, throwing away foods that are expired or are stale.
- Eat anything that was saved as a leftover within 24-hours or throw it away.
- Cut down on the overall fat consumption per day, focusing on minimizing saturated fats.
- Minimize your intake of salts, especially focusing on the salt added to your food already.
- Do not drink more than one alcoholic drink per day, if at all.

Foods that have been found to help reduce inflammation include:

- Oily fish found in cold water, such as herring, mackerel, tuna, and salmon.
- Berries, especially those that are dark in color like blackberries and blueberries.
- Nuts from trees, such as cashews, hazelnuts, almonds, and walnuts.This excludes peanuts, which is more of a legume or found on the ground.
- Seeds like pumpkin and sunflower seeds.
- Whole grains like whole wheat and whole oats.
- Dark green and leafy vegetables like kale and spinach.
- Soy foods like tofu and soy milk
- Tempeh
- Dairy products that are low fat.
- Any kind of pepper, such as jalapeno or bell pepper.
- Mushrooms and various fungi
- Beets
- Tomatoes
- Turmeric
- Ginger, both fresh and ground.
- Garlic
- Olive oils
- Cherries that are fresh and tart, not maraschino cherries.

- Dark chocolate, over 70% cocoa.

- Fresh herbs, like basil and cilantro.

- Fresh, cracked black pepper.

In addition to the suggestions above on how to start your planning process, below is a plan for reducing your inflammation through your diet and lifestyle. This may be what you consider a "complete" plan that you will want to work into. A word of caution and reminder; make choices that are realistic to your life as it is now and avoids actions and choices that you know will harm your unique makeup. If you are allergic to certain foods or know you have a sensitivity to them, but they are listed on the foods list above or in a suggestion below, then do not feel required to follow it. Make this plan customized to your needs with your focus always on improving your health and well-being. With this focus in mind, the plan you develop is sure to be great for you!

The "Complete" Anti-Inflammatory Action Plan

1. Remove the junk foods and processed foods from your kitchen, pantry, work drawers, and life. Keep tabs on the ingredient labels for anything that comes pre-packaged to

make sure what you are eating is actually healthy and not just junk food in disguise.

2. Stick to whole foods when you can. You may not always be able to choose a whole food because life is busy and hectic, but plan ahead for times when this may or will happen. For example, instead of buying a pastry and a fancy coffee on your way to work in the morning, prep something that will support your healthy living the night before so you can still grab-and-go but without the negative health consequences (and added expense!).

3. Increase the amount of fruit you eat every day. This can be fresh, canned or frozen, but make sure if it is not fresh that there is no added sugar or ingredients to it. Fruit juice does not really count because it loses a lot of the necessary nutrients whole versions contain.

4. Increase the number of vegetables you eat every day. These can also be fresh, canned or frozen like the fruits. They also should not have any added sugars or ingredients if they are packaged. Some people simply do not like the taste of vegetables. That is ok! Try to get some in on a daily basis in a minimally processed way. Find a few that you can eat often, and if necessary, get a couple of servings in through soups, smoothies, or juice.

5. Focus on whole grains for each meal. Sometimes rice and whole wheat toast can get a little "old" for your taste

buds. There are so many options out there that it can be fun to experiment a little. Look for some different options at the store like wild rice, couscous, teff, Kamut, quinoa, buckwheat, faro, and millet. Try to make it a fun challenge to find different ways to prepare these various ingredients.

6. Eat oily, cold-water fish twice per week. Look for fish that are wild-caught or sustainably sourced.

7. Increase your intake of additional protein or omega-3 fatty acid sources, including chia seeds, flax seeds, hemp seeds, edamame, or walnuts.

8. Cut back on your caffeine consumption to two cups per day. A cup is equal to eight ounces.

9. When drinking something other than water, choose teas like rooibos, white or green or black coffee.

10. Carry a snack bag of mixed, raw, whole nuts and seeds to snack on throughout the day.

11. Snack on olives throughout the day to make sure you get plenty of "good" fat in your diet.

12. Swap out your cooking oils for either avocado oil or extra virgin olive oil.

13. Cut out foods that contain any refined sugar that is added to it. The nutrition label provides this information to help you determine if the sugar in the item is from added refined sugar sources or natural sweeteners. The

ingredient list is currently necessary for this information, but soon it will be easily distinguished on the label under the "sugar" line.

14. Cut back on trans-fats. There are key terms in the ingredient list of packaged foods that are "red flags," and mean that you need to avoid that food. For example, stay away from anything that says, "partially hydrogenated oil," or "hydrogenated oil."

15. Increase your physical activity. This does not mean you have to start running or working out at a gym. This may mean that you get up and take a walk around your floor a couple of times a day, or park further away from your front door. Find ways to sneak in more physical activity during your day, even if it is in small spurts.

16. Make sure you get plenty of sleep every night. Try to develop a good night time routine that helps you fall asleep and stay asleep for about seven to nine hours every night. And make it quality sleep if you can! This helps you function better the next day, but also helps your body restore itself throughout the evening. Just one night of lost hours of sleep can inflame your cells and start damaging your tissue. Create a plan to help you avoid this at all costs.

17. Focus on reducing constant stress in your life every day. Things like deep breathing or meditation are excellent

tools to help you calm your body down and deal with stress. Stress can harm your body and mind, especially if it is chronic stress. It is important that you create a plan to deal with the stresses of daily life as well as the big things that happen that can derail all your hard work.

How to Start and Maintain Your Plan

Again, the best way to implement this anti-inflammatory action plan is to tackle one item at a time with a realistic set of steps. It is a gradual process that can help you move into this lifestyle with confidence and success. This gradual approach is what will make your plan start with success and continue it for the long-term. Each time you make an empowered, sustainable step forward, you keep moving down your path to an anti-inflamed, healthy, and happy life. Some people may be able to adopt this plan in a few weeks while others may take more than six months to develop a full plan for themselves. Do not focus on what someone else is doing, but rather on what will work for you.

And just because you do not see an immediate change does not mean it is not working. Each positive choice you make compounds with the other positive choice you continue to make, setting off a ripple of healing and supportive actions inside your body. You may not see or feel them yet, but you must trust that they are working in your favor. Eventually, you will see a trimmer waist or experience more energy or even enjoy the minimization of illnesses, but you must give it time to work!

An Anti-Inflammatory Guide for Groceries

Fresh Foods:

Organic vegetables such as Brussels sprouts, broccoli, bok choy, beets, asparagus, collard greens, kale, kelp, nori, spinach, swiss chard, sweet potatoes, and zucchini. Other vegetables to consider include cauliflower, onions, asparagus, carrots, cucumber, leeks, sprouts, and peas.

Organic fruit such as raspberries, blueberries, blackberries, avocado, plums, cherries, and apples.

Organic protein sources such as turkey, chicken, eggs, peas, lentils, legumes, oily fish, and beans.

Stick to the outer edges of most grocery stores to find whole and fresh foods to stock your fridge and pantry. Most fruits and vegetables found in the produce section of the store are good choices to add to your anti-inflammatory diet.

Pantry Staples:

Additional protein sources from protein powders or dry beans and lentils.

Whole grains such as brown, black, red or wild rice, millet, quinoa, buckwheat, and couscous.

Selection of beverages such as seltzer water, unsweetened teas with minimal caffeine, and black coffee.

Various oils such as walnut, sesame, hemp seed, flax seed, coconut, avocado, and extra virgin olive oil.

Seeds and nuts that are unsalted and raw such as pumpkin seeds, chia seeds, flax seeds, hemp seeds, sesame seeds, walnuts, almonds, cashews, macadamia nuts, sunflower seeds, and tahini.

Natural sweeteners such as pure maple syrup (not corn syrup that has been colored), organic and raw honey, and stevia extract.

Condiments such as nut butter (not peanut), cocoa powder with no added sugars or ingredients, whole peppercorns, sea salt, various spices, various dry herbs, and apple cider vinegar.

Always read ingredient labels for foods that are packaged and prepared for you. Look for minimal ingredient lists, try to choose organic options, and stay away from trigger words like "hydrogenated." In addition, when you are first starting out finding brands and reading labels, it can be overwhelming looking in depth at all your choices. Start by shopping mostly in the organic or health-food aisles found in most grocery stores to minimize the selection and increase your chances of finding anti-inflammatory packaged foods.

Chapter 4: What is an Anti-Inflammatory Diet?

Inflammation plays an important role in your body, but the difference between "good" and "bad" inflammation can sometimes be confused. There is "good" inflammation. This is the natural reaction that your body goes through to help heal and protect you from influences that can harm your well-being. The problem is when inflammation is triggered and continues to occur. This is called "Chronic" inflammation,and this kind of "bad" inflammation is what causes negative health side effects. It is possible to suffer from inflammation for a couple of weeks to several years. The longer and more severed the chronic inflammation, the more serious the side effects can be for you. It can even lead to death! Luckily for you, there are several steps you can take to minimize the amount of inflammation in your body so that you support and improve your overall health.

When your body is injured, infected, or is ill inflammation jumps in to save that day. In fact, the purpose of inflammation is to prevent these things from occurring or minimize the effect something like this could have on your body if it was unprotected. White blood cells are triggered in response to an "outside" invader or influence that threatens the balance of your body. In addition to the white blood cells, your inflammation response produces immune cells and other substances like cytokines all to help ward off infection. When inflammation first occurs, you can often feel and see the response in your body. The area of injury or infection can become painful, warm, or red. But when inflammation is constant, it may not be as obvious. And when inflammation is silently attacking your own body as if it were a foreigner invader, you create an opportunity for serious diseases such as cancer, fatty liver disease, heart issues, and type-2 diabetes.

If you suffer from obesity or constant stress in your life chances are that you also suffer from chronic inflammation. The habits you reenact every day are one of the best determining factors for the likelihood of chronic inflammation in your body. The way you live your life and eat foods determine most cases of chronic inflammation in the United States. The Western diet is high in things like high-fructose corn syrup and refined sugars, both of which are known inflammation instigators for extended periods of time. "Empty" carbs and processed foods are also linked to chronic inflammation and prevalent in the American diet. Eating these foods often have been linked over and over again in scientific studies to the increased risk of developing insulin resistance, type-2 diabetes, and obesity. More studies have shown a link between carbs and processed foods to chronic inflammation. Other inflammation culprits include a sedentary lifestyle, use of tobacco, and overuse of alcohol.

Your diet is one of the best methods for reducing inflammation in your body, and it is one of the easiest (and cheapest) methods you can control. Some foods have been linked to the reduction of inflammation while others are known to exacerbate the problems you are experiencing. The general rule in any diet designed to help reduce inflammation is to eat more foods that you know will help fight inflammation and stay away as often as possible from the foods that are known to cause it. This means eating more whole foods on a daily basis and staying away from refined or processed foods. To go even further, consider choosing whole foods that also give you a dose of antioxidants to help fight off and reduce the number of free radicals bouncing around in your body. Free radicals, like inflammation, are a natural response to support your well-being, but when they are not controlled and limited, they can lead to a variety of health issues. One of the most dangerous health concerns of excessive free radicals is the increase in chronic inflammation. Foods with a lot of antioxidants help naturally control your level of free radicals, and a lot of these foods are found in most anti-inflammatory meal plans. What makes an anti-inflammatory diet different than other options, like a low-carb diet, is that it supports proper nutrition that your body needs for optimal functioning. It is not about losing weight, but rather gaining your health back. Anti-inflammatory diets mix in antioxidant-rich foods through "good" fats, proteins, and carbs in every meal and snack. You also will focus on proper vitamins, minerals, fiber, and water consumption. It is considered a lifestyle, meaning most anti-inflammatory diet plans include recommendations for not just eating, but sleep and physical activity as well.

Recommendations for How to Follow an Anti-Inflammatory Lifestyle

To truly change and live a healthy life, you need to change more than just the food that you eat. The extra things you do are what assist you in reaching and maintaining your goals. The following list is full of recommendations for living and loving the life of anti-inflammation:

- Sleep well each night. Your well-being is directly impacted by the amount and the quality of sleep you get each evening. The time you take to rest your mind and body at night is the time your body takes to inventory itself and reboot your system. This period of rest is also the time your body begins to naturally reduce inflammation that you do not need. If you do not allow your body to take this important time, you slow down and can even stop the process. It does not matter how well you are doing regarding the food you are putting into your body, if you do not give it the chance to heal at night, you are just spinning your wheels, metaphorically speaking.
- Make your body work often. Every day you need to move your body moderately for approximately 20 minutes.

Notice this says "move your body," and not "exercise." You do not need to go for a run or lift weights to check this off your to-do list every day. Instead, you need to do things like walk for five minutes after dinner or parking further away,so you have to walk a long distance to work or home. Breaking up the 20 minutes into five-minute intervals is an easy way to sneak in your daily requirement. When you begin to do this, you also help reduce the risk of various diseases along with inflammation.

- Take supplements when needed, especially if you are having trouble figuring out your meals. When you begin changing what you eat it can be overwhelming. You need to balance carbs, proteins, fats, minerals, vitamins, etc. and that is a lot to tackle, especially if you have never done it before. To help you make empowered choices and to silence the negative voices, consider adding a supplement to your daily routine. This way you know you are getting the nutrients you need until you figure out your plate. A good multi-vitamin is great for the transition period you will go through when learning about foods you like and that work well together to give you a nice balanced meal full of all the good stuff you need. In addition, you can add in supplements like curcumin and omega-3 fatty acids to make sure you get these in your diet until you figure out whole food sources. It is important to recognize that supplements are not intended to be something you take for the long term or as a permanent part of your health plan. They are simply a transitional tool until you find your plan that fulfills all your dietary needs through whole foods. Supplements can have a place during the big changes, but make sure to "retire" them when you get a handle on your foods.

When you do make the change to the anti-inflammatory diet, a host of benefits accompany the feeling of empowerment and health. A sample of the benefits you can potentially enjoy are:

1. Improved energy levels and mood.
2. Better triglyceride, blood sugar, and cholesterol levels.
3. Reduced markers in your blood for inflammation.
4. Lowered obesity, heart disease, type-2 diabetes, depression, and cancer risk for development.
5. Enhanced treatment for diseases like autoimmune diseases.This includes arthritis, lupus, and irritable bowel syndrome.

To generalize the results, chronic inflammation is significantly reduced when you change your lifestyle to support anti-inflammation, including changing your diet. This lowered chronic inflammation is what helps lower the risk of developing additional serious diseases as well as help heal others you may already be suffering from. Inflammation is the result of your diet, lifestyle, and environment. When you change up these key areas of your like to control your well-being and health, you can expect to see a big difference. Unfortunately, the Western diet is dominated by unhealthy food choices and relationships. This means that Americans and those that eat a Western diet are more at risk than other cultures for developing chronic inflammation. Men are also at more of a risk than women are. Chronic inflammation is directly linked to heart disease, which is currently the number one killer in the United States. By changing the quality of your like and making good choices regarding your body's nutritional intake, you take great steps in lengthening your life span and the quality of that life.

The "How" of the Anti-inflammatory Diet

The focus of this lifestyle is on plants. It encourages you to consume mostly plants that offer specific chemicals that are known to reduce the body's inflammation levels naturally. The reason this diet focuses on plants is that of their organic ability to produce various beneficial chemicals for the human body. One of the chemicals most plants produce that is so good for your body is called phytochemicals. These are important chemicals for plant function, and while certain phytochemicals are poisonous for the human body, others are vital. For example, you most likely can name several plants that you recognize should be eaten regularly, while there are specific berries or mushrooms you know you need to be cautious of in the wild because they can be dangerous to your health if you eat them. Because of the amazing natural abilities of plants to thrive and protect themselves with these phytochemicals, you should not be caught off guard when you learn that these plants that you can eat safely are some of the best foods you can eat.

This natural protections from plants for your organs and cells is what makes the anti-inflammatory diet so unique. Many contemporary diet plans encourage whole foods and a plant focus, but while they may avoid the subject of inflammation, most of the time the benefits they list for consuming these foods is because of their anti-inflammatory properties. The protection these plants offer to your body against all levels of chronic inflammation is vital to your overall health and longevity.

Yes, not all inflammation should be counteracted. When you are fighting a cold or ingest a toxin, inflammation is a natural response you need to rely upon If you have an injury, damaged cells send out a specific chemical to your blood vessels so fluid can be leaked into the tissue around the injury site. The swelling of the tissue is what protects the body from a spreading injury and also provides an isolated space for the damaged area to heal. The swelling side effect alerts your immune system that the area requires specific cells that need to clean up the damaged cells or even to come in and kill the infected cells. It is when your body sends inflammation-triggering cells to locations that do not heal, or tissue is swollen and inflamed for a long time that your body begins to malfunction. This is when more diseases can manifest in the body,and you are no longer equipped to fight them off. You are too busy fighting yourself!

The majority of the research published discusses the footprints or biomarkers of the body's inflammation. Some of these "footprints" include C-reactive proteins, or CRP, and cytokines. These are chemicals that travel in your bloodstream and act as a sort of signaling device for inflammation that is occurring in the body. Foods that are known to lower these markers are also known as anti-inflammatory foods. The markers are lower from eating these foods because the chronic inflammation in your body is lower. When you lower your inflammation, you lower your risk of developing a variety of deadly and painful diseases. Some doctors may still consider the positive effects the anti-inflammatory diet has on inflammation as "controversial," but no doctor can deny that a healthy diet can positively impact your overall health, including lowering your inflammation and risk of certain diseases. And the anti-inflammatory diet definitely is a lifestyle that falls in the "healthy" category!

When you are choosing foods for your anti-inflammatory diet plan, make sure you are selecting foods for their properties associated with lowering inflammation rather than because they have a specific nutrient in them that are known to lower inflammation. You want to choose foods that are going to give you the most "bang for your buck." You want foods that are going to support your body and satisfy your hunger and taste buds. This requires you to choose foods that contain a high level of healthy fat and beneficial phytochemicals, are plant-based and are whole food.

Beans, nuts, whole grains, and specific spices and herbs are a few of the primary foods you want to consume. These types of foods should not alarm you; they are the food types that often make the top of most healthy eating diet plans. Another healthy chemical that these foods offer is called "flavonoids." This is a compound found in many plant-based foods that are known for helping lower inflammation levels. Other chemicals that certain foods offer to help lower inflammation are omega-3 fatty acids, often found in oily fish, and fiber. And while these foods perform wonders for your health and the number you see on the scale, they are not magic pills that will have you dropping several dress sizes overnight while curing all your ailments. You have to give these healthy foods a chance to work their magic. This means adopting and sticking to the anti-inflammatory diet for an extended period of timein order to truly enjoy the benefits it has to offer you.

The Mediterranean Diet - A Good Example of Eating to Lower Inflammation

Not all diets or meal plans fit all people, but there are a few dietary guidelines that are good for almost every person and definitely worth considering. Any adaptation of the anti-inflammatory diet fits this description, but the "Mediterranean Diet," is a commonly mentioned anti-inflammatory plan you should look into. The foundational principles rest in the anti-inflammatory guidelines for healthy eating, but also specify the types and frequency of consuming various fish. In addition, it gives you room to enjoy a little wine, too! If it works for you and your life, when you follow the diet based off the cultures living along the Mediterranean Sea, you can have a small glass of red wine a day and still be "following the rules!"

All anti-inflammatory diets introduce the foundational concepts of avoiding pro-inflammation foods like unhealthy fats and refined foods while consuming a large number of anti-inflammatory foods like fruits, vegetables, fish, and whole grains. The presentation and preparation of these foods are what makes each one distinct. A significant part of this includes the size of the portions during each meal. In most anti-inflammatory diets, including the Mediterranean Diet, portion sizes are very specific. You will learn more about this later in the book.

The primary components of the Mediterranean Diet are:

- Meals are a social event and should be enjoyed in the company of friends and family often. This also includes the preparation and clean up of a meal.
- Pour yourself a small glass of red wine a few times a week. Drinking red wine in moderation is approved on the Mediterranean Diet, but you do not have to do this if you do not want to or should not drink alcohol at all.
- Two times a week make sure you eat lean poultry and oily fish.
- If you must eat red meat, do not eat it more than two times a month. Try not to eat it at all!
- Season your food with spices and various herbs instead of other, unhealthy seasoning options.
- Choose healthy fats, like extra virgin olive oil, over unhealthy options, like butter.

When you follow an anti-inflammatory diet like this, you do not have to give up alcohol or bread completely, but you do have to consume them in moderation and with empowerment. Sometimes you will be advised against these "treats" altogether, while others will be more lenient on your consumption of them. Make sure you listen to your body and your team of professionals, as well as allow yourself the permission to eat with empowerment.

Chapter 5: Stocking Your Kitchen

The best way to keep eating easy and healthy is to stock your fridge, freezer, and pantry with whole foods known to help reduce your inflammation. The following chapter is designed to help you learn what some healthy foods you can keep on hand at all times.

Healing your body and supporting your overall well-being is best done through your diet, but you will have a hard time doing that if your kitchen is always full of pro-inflammatory foods. Not only does this provide unnecessary temptation, but it also makes it hard to plan out what you are going to eat if you have to weed through unhealthy options that you have on hand. In addition, planning out your bigger meals for the week can also make it easier for you when the time is short,and schedules are busy. Adopting these habits of meal planning and clean stocking means you always have a healthy option at your fingertips.

But before you get into the in's and out's of organizing your food storage, give yourself time to switch everything over. You do not need to completely overhaul your pantry and fridge at one time. Thinking of it this way can become soul-crushing and ridiculously expensive. It is a sure way to set yourself up for a negative experience and a definite loss. A different approach is to replace things as they run out with a healthier option. This means that when your sugar bag is empty, you choose a less refined sweetener that you can turn to. Or when your bags of chips are gone, you pick up dried fruits and vegetables for a crunchy snack instead. As the entire process of adopting an anti-inflammatory diet, it is best to do this one step at a time. And make sure to celebrate each step of the way!

Get Your Groceries Here!

You can get almost all of your meats, produce, and perishables from stores like Whole Foods, Thrive Market online, and Amazon, which is excellent for your dry goods, especially if you choose "Subscribe and Save." Your local co-op or farmer's market is also good to shop at, especially for local and organic foods, but you can still get a few staples at your regular grocery store as well. To avoid having to make multiple trips at various stores, try to use their delivery service is available, or shop through a grocery delivery service like Instacart. These services typically cost a small fee for use but can save you a bunch of time and headache depending on your schedule and requirements. The more you replace items with healthy alternatives, the more opportunity you have to try different brands and find the best stores with the best prices. Give it time to refine your grocery stores, too.

Finally, healthier foods are almost always more expensive than their conventional options. If you are concerned about price, make sure to always choose organic for the "Dirty Dozen" foods, but be more lenient with other options if you need to. The "Dirty Dozen list includes foods that are almost always contaminated with pesticides or grown from GMO, or "Genetically Modified Organism," seeds unless you choose the organic option. The list is as follows:

1. Strawberries
2. Spinach
3. Nectarines
4. Apples
5. Grapes
6. Peaches
7. Cherries
8. Pears
9. Tomatoes
10. Celery
11. Potatoes
12. Sweet bell peppers

What Should Be in Your Fridge

- Produce that is seasonal and organic. Produce is the staple of the anti-inflammatory diet. Making sure you eat a variety of vegetables and fruit on a daily basis is crucial to your health. This is why you need to always have full produce drawers in your fridge. And keep it rotating; try not to keep the same foods in there, because the seasons do change, and so should your produce! But also, because keeping it different bits of help keep your taste buds happy. That being said, try to always keep some sort of leafy green available for a salad base, such as spinach, kale, or lettuces. From there, you can have a variety of anything else, including a selection of fresh herbs, such as basil, mint, or parsley.

- Eggs that are pasture-raised and organic. When you think breakfast, eggs are an easy staple. Of course, you can eat eggs any time of day,and a hard-boiled egg is a great go-to snack for the afternoon. You can usually find a local farmer who sells organic eggs from pasture-raised chickens, but if you do not have good options, look for Vital Farms eggs, which of organic eggs from a certified humane farm that allows their hens to roam free in a pasture.

- Meats that are pasture-raised and organic. Just like the eggs, you should try to choose lean meats that are raised in humane and organic settings. Grass-fed is ideal. Meats from these sources are not only healthier for you but are also better for the environment. Keep lean meats to a minimum during the week, ideally no more than four times. For the other nights, choose fish proteins and eat vegetarian for at least one day. When you do eat meats, look for chicken breasts that still have their skin and bones, bone-in pork chops or shoulder, flank steaks, and lamb, chick, or turkey ground meat. If you have trouble finding a good source of high-quality meat in your area, look for online services like Butcher Box.

- Milk made from non-dairy sources. When at home, it is a good practice to avoid dairy ingredients. This helps cut back on your dairy intake throughout the day. When you want to make a smoothie or put a little "milk" in your coffee, adding a splash of organic almond or coconut milk is a great and healthy alternative. If you cannot find a milk alternative that you like, consider buying raw milk from a local farmer. Look for farmers that allow their cows to roam in the pasture and are fed grass. This also applies to butter and ghee. Look for organic sources that are pasture-fed.

- Coconut water that is minimally processed. Sometimes you want a little something more than filtered water. You can add this to smoothies or juice. Make sure the brand you choose is not developed from concentrate or have additional flavors or sugars. Coconut water not s like a vacation in a glass, but it is also a good source of electrolytes.

- Other beverages to keep on hand, if you prefer include carbonated water and kombucha. Kombucha provides a nice tang and carbonation. In addition, it is also very good for your gut health. If you are not a fan of the taste of kombucha, you can find a good alternative to carbonated drinks with carbonated waters. A squeeze of lime or a few pieces of fresh fruit in your sparkling water can be a very refreshing treat.

- Red wine. Most alcohol tends to inflame your body, but a few glasses a couple of times a week of good quality and organic wine is a great way to close out your evening or week. Choose a full-bodied red wine to enjoy most of the nutrients in the grapes used to make the vintage.

- Apple cider vinegar is organic and raw. This ingredient is great for a variety of recipes, including making skin care products and other crafts that should not be eaten. You can add this to salad dressings or just drink it straight. For those that do not like the taste of vinegar but want the health benefits, shooting an ounce of this in the morning can help support your gut health and balance your hormones, and then you can chase it with a cup of coffee or kombucha.

- Gluten-free, whole wheat bread. It does not need to be gluten-free if you are not sensitive to gluten, but when you are choosing a loaf of bread to keep on hand, choose a simple carbohydrate that will do the best for your overall health goals. This type of bread makes a good base for a sandwich or toast for breakfast and is hearty,so you only need to eat one or two slices at a time to be filled.

- Hard cheeses and meats that have been cured. A good block of Parmigiano Reggiano is good to have on hand for shredding over salads or other dishes. Other hard cheeses in a block form are also nice to have on hand for a quick snack or nice appetizer to serve when company is over. A selection of cured meats, like salami or prosciutto, are also good to have in stock for a nice protein boost.

- Various condiments. Almost all premade condiments contain ingredients you want to avoid. This includes things like ketchup and salad dressings. Instead, consider making your own. Salad dressings are particularly easy at making and storing. But when you are out of time or out of steam, look for brands that are the cleanest, like Primal Kitchen or Tessemae. If you want flavor and spice, have a selection of hot sauces. These are a great way to add flavor without a lot of additives. The same goes for salsa and tomato paste. You can also find cleaner brands for things like mayonnaise and ketchup. Tub of hummus is also a nice condiment for dipping carrot and celery sticks into.

What Should Be in Your Freezer

- Vegetables and fruits that are frozen. Try to stock your freezer with a variety of organic vegetables and fruits. You can purchase pre-packaged versions in the store, or freeze your own. These work great for making smoothies at home or to add flavor to water. Vegetables can be added to soups and stir-fry's easily from your freezer in a pinch. The benefit of buying a package is that the vegetable or fruit is often picked when it is in season and frozen at its peak of freshness. This means that when you consume it, it most likely has the most nutrients, sometimes even more so than fresh varieties in the store. Great fruit options to stock in your freezer include all types of berries, bananas, pineapple, and mango. Great vegetables to have in your freezer include butternut squash, green beans, and peas.

- Smoothie packs. Like frozen fruit, these packets are a nice thing to always have on hand, if you like smoothies. These little pre-packaged goods offer a host of different fruits and sometimes vegetables mixed together so you can easily whip up a tasty frozen drink. Some packets also include super-fruits like Acai and turmeric, both known for their anti-inflammatory properties. These are not essential to a well-stocked kitchen but can make a big difference in your routine if you enjoy smoothies often.

- Leaves from Kaffir limes. If you are a fan of Asian cuisine, especially Thai foods, you should always have a few of these leaves on hand. They are a vibrant and fresh flavor you can add to anything from marinade to soup.

- Knobs of pre-peeled ginger. You may need to do the leg work of preparing the ginger for the freezer yourself, but when you are in need of ginger in a meal,and your fresh knob of ginger is out, these frozen back-ups will save you. Freezing prepared ginger chunks that are about one inch in size can help make sure you always keep a stock of this tasty and anti-inflammatory ingredient on hand. You also do not need to thaw ginger before you use it in a recipe. Simply grate the frozen knob with a microplane to add the flavor to the recipe or dish.

- Wheatgrass. You can keep the actual grass frozen or buy powder and store it in your freezer. This sweet light green ingredient is an excellent addition to a smoothie or soup. Make sure the brand you purchase is organic to ensure you get the most nutrients from your food. If you have never considered it before, it is time to do more research on the benefits of wheatgrass. It is a rich source of minerals and vitamins as well as things like chlorophyll for its healing properties.

- Organic and wild-caught seafood. If you are worried about the cost of purchasing fresh, organic, wild-caught, sustainably-sourced seafood, go over to the freezer section and look at what is available there. You can usually find a bag or box of suitable fish that is a lesser price than the fresh version. And having a frozen stash of appropriate seafood means you have a better chance of getting your two servings a week. Some easy options to keep on hand include shrimp and salmon. Other excellent choices that you can find often include tuna and halibut.

- Bone broth made from scratch or store-bought organic versions. It is best to make your own broth to monitor what is going into the pot, but if you cannot or do not want to make your own, look for a clean brand that you can stash in your freezer to sip on during a cold evening or use as a base for soups.

Chapter 6: Anti-Inflammatory 2-Week Meal Plan and Recipes for Life

When you follow the meal plan below for the next two weeks, you will follow a meal plan intended to reset your body and habits. It is not intended to be a strict and unrealistic plan, but rather a guide for healing your body in a nourishing and healthy manner. As you dive deeper into the anti-inflammatory lifestyle, you will divefurther into these recipes to alter them to fit your fitness and health goals' however, as you begin your journey, this is a great place to begin.

As you begin your healthy eating plan, it is important to remember the basics of the anti-inflammatory diet plan. When you are considering the anti-inflammatory diet, there are a few questions you will consider: do you need this diet, what foods can you eat, and what can you eat to help reduce your inflammation? If you need to be on this diet is dependent on your own health needs. If you know you are struggling with some form of chronic inflammation, you should be seriously considering the anti-inflammatory diet.

As you begin your anti-inflammatory meal plan, you need to start in the right frame of mind. First, you need to be focused on foods that are going to offer the most anti-inflammatory and nutritional boost to your diet. As you refocus on these foods, you need to let go of other foods like gluten-rich and processed foods. The following meal plan and recipes are provided to give you a starting point and a few resources to rotate on a regular basis. You can follow the plan exactly or rotate the plan and recipes according to your needs and preferences. You can browse through the recipe guide for alternatives to the suggestions in the meal plan as well if you want.

The following recipes are designed to give you a healthy dose of "super foods" or anti-inflammatory foods in your daily diet. The foods and recipes include a variety of fatty acids, minerals, soluble fiber, prebiotics, and vitamins in your nutritional intake. The idea behind this two-week meal plan is to give you enough energy and support to find your way back to a balanced body. Once you master this dietary process, you can begin to address your other lifestyle habits that will support or detract from your anti-inflammatory lifestyle.

The Two-Week Anti-inflammatory Diet Plan

The following diet plan includes suggestions for healthy breakfasts, lunches, dinners, and snacks. In addition, some alternative beverages are introduced, other than water and coffee.

Day 1:

Breakfast: Morning muffins made with ginger, apple, and rhubarb. Ginger adds a nice zing to the breakfast food as well as offers a good dose of anti-inflammatory agents. The recipe is also free from dairy and gluten, making it a great choice for many dietary plans.

Lunch: Pumpkin soup. Pumpkin provides a lot of anti-inflammatory support in the form of beta-cryptoxanthin. To properly absorb this agent, you need the healthy fats found in this recipe. Make sure you select a high-quality source of pumpkin with strong skins. Cooking the soup with skins on makes this recipe even easier for you!

Dinner: Brown rice topped with stir-fried chili peppers, tofu, and Chinese cabbage. The fresh ginger in this recipe offers you more of that anti-inflammatory benefits, along with a good source of protein in the tofu. Additionally, the whole grain brown rice and chili peppers are great ingredients to support your anti-inflammatory needs.

Snack: one cup of mixed, raw seeds and nuts

Day 2:

Breakfast: Porridge topped with dehydrated cherries. Whole grain oats or porridge sprinkled on top with dehydrated cherries provides a good serving of the antioxidant anthocyanin.

Lunch: Salad with winter fruits and a pomegranate and agave vinaigrette dressing. A bowl full of mixed greens topped with grapes, pears, and persimmons is a beautiful way to freshen up your lunchtime. Drizzle the salad with the dressing just before eating; otherwise, the fruit becomes too soft when it sits in the vinaigrette for a length of time.

Dinner: Snapper and spinach served with a side of herbs and rice. Snapper is a good fish to get a serving of omega-3 fatty acids that you need for fighting inflammation. The spinach offers a good source of anti-inflammatory benefits, too. Served with the side of whole grain rice helps keep you full,and the fresh herbs add a nice aroma and flavor.

Snack: One cup of mixed, raw seeds and nuts

Day 3:

Breakfast: Barley served with a poached egg, wilted spinach, sliced avocado, and sautéed mushrooms. Eggs are a good source of protein and when consumed in moderation are good healthy fat, too. The avocado also offers an excellent source of healthy fat, as well as other anti-inflammatory benefits.

Lunch: Potato and smoked salmon tartine with a side salad and vinaigrette. The salmon offers a good amount of omega-3 fatty acid and the leafy green salad provides additional anti-inflammatory support. If you want something a little more filling, consider trading the salad for a soup that also supports anti-inflammation.

Dinner: Poached egg and curry potatoes with a side salad and vinaigrette.This is a simple dinner that you can make over and over. It is sure to fill you up and help you fight off inflammation. If poached eggs are not in your skill set or you do not like the taste, try cooking them in a skillet or boiling them to slice over the potatoes. Remember, eggs should come from a sustainable farm,and the chickens that they come from should be free-range. This makes sure you have the best serving of anti-inflammatory omega-3 fatty acids.

Snack: Plain yogurt mixed with cinnamon and topped with fresh fruit. The yogurt offers a good source of protein, gut support, and additional anti-inflammatory benefits. The cinnamon is a good flavoring that works double to help you fight off inflammation. You can choose whatever fruit you want to top your yogurt with, but berries give a little extra anti-inflammatory boost to your snack.

Day 4:

Breakfast: Herbed tomatoes and beans spread over whole-grain toast. Beans are one of the best plant-based protein sources and a good ingredient to fill you up. The tomatoes offer a nice tang and liquid to your whole grain serving.

Lunch: Steamed salmon and a halved avocado served over a cup and a half of sauerkraut with a side salad and vinaigrette. Suaerkraut is an excellent fermented food that helps stabilize your GI tract. Make sure to drizzle extra virgin olive oil over the salmon and salad to provide another source of healthy fat and anti-inflammatory benefits to your meal.

Dinner: Red bell peppers stuffed with Italian filling. A twist on the classic stuffed pepper, this version chooses the red bell because of its beta carotene and vitamin C content. The additional ingredients provide their own health support and anti-inflammatory benefits.

Snack: Mixed salad greens drizzled with extra virgin olive oil and balsamic vinegar. Choose high-quality vinegar to add to your salad. Not only will this enhance the taste but you will get more benefits from this ingredient when chosen for quality over price.

Day 5:

Prepare dinner in the morning so that it is ready in the evening.

Breakfast: Sautéed spinach and scrambled eggs over a cup of brown rice. Adding the power of the whole grain rice with the antioxidants in spinach and protein of eggs is a surefire way of starting your morning on the right foot.

Lunch: Slices of sushi-grade salmon and tuna with cooked edamame and a small cup of miso soup or organic bone broth. This slightly Asian lunch is light but powerful. The fresh fish is tasty and clean. Make sure you choose fish from a reliable seafood seller and that it is wild caught, rather than farmed. This helps to ensure you get the most benefits from the protein source.

Dinner: Make sure to start this in the morning! A hot bowl of chili on a cool evening or when you have been rushing around all day is a nice way to end the business. The recipe does call for salt, which can cause you to retain water and exacerbate inflammation symptoms. If you react to salt, cut down the amount in the recipe and consider adding in spices or hot peppers to add flavor without the additive. You should also make sure you select beans that are canned in low- or no-sodium cans or cook them from a dried state. If you want to add something on top, consider raw pumpkin seeds, slices of avocado or a dollop of plain Greek yogurt.

Snack: Slices of vegetables to dip into guacamole or hummus.

Day 6:

Breakfast: Crepes filled with slices of banana and strawberry. The recipe in this book is easy and gluten-free. You can add a few dark chocolate nibs (70% or higher cocoa content!) or a dollop of vanilla Greek yogurt for some added taste, texture, and anti-inflammation fighting, if you want.

Lunch: Mixed greens topped with chopped tomatoes, roasted vegetables, and chickpeas. Chickpeas are a nice addition to the salad, providing you with anti-inflammatory agents as well as flavor. If you need dressing, drizzle a little extra virgin olive oil and balsamic vinegar over top.

Dinner: "Burgers" made from black beans and sweet potatoes and served on bibb lettuce leaves. Dress your burger with toppings like sliced tomatoes, avocado, and red onion. Sprinkle a few sprouts on the top for extra help for your digestion. The sweet potato added to the "burger" mix brings beta carotene and vitamin C that supports your health and fights back inflammation.

Snack: Plain yogurt mixed with cinnamon and topped with fresh fruit. The yogurt offers a good source of protein, gut support, and additional anti-inflammatory benefits. The cinnamon is a good flavoring that works double to help you fight off inflammation. You can choose whatever fruit you want to top your yogurt with, but berries give a little extra anti-inflammatory boost to your snack.

Day 7:

Breakfast: Two slices of whole wheat toast spread with mashed avocado and topped with slices of smoked salmon. This combination contains immense flavor and a variety of textures. It also gives you several anti-inflammatory benefits, as well.

Lunch:Red bell peppers stuffed with quinoa and ground turkey. Another twist to the popular stuffed pepper recipe. Quinoa is a superfood as well as filling,and the ground turkey offers a lean protein source inside the sweet pepper "bowl." The red pepper offers the best source of nutrients and a sweeter taste than other peppers, like a green bell pepper.

Dinner: Steamed green beans served alongside mashed sweet potato and baked trout. Trout is a tasty fish full of omega-3 fatty acid and protein. Consider this your second serving of fish for the week!

Snack: One cup of mixed, raw seeds and nuts

Day 8:

Breakfast: Blueberry and raspberry smoothie. When you are on the run in the morning, a smoothie packed full of fruit and vegetables is a great option. You can prepare the ingredients ahead of time,so all you have to do is through the contents into a blender and mix up before you head out the door. You can also pre-mix the smoothie and keep it in the refrigerator for an even faster "escape" out the door.

Lunch: Shredded carrot and cabbage "slaw" topped with stir-fry tofu. Shredding these super vegetables offers a bright base for your taste-loaded tofu. If you do not like the slaw raw, consider adding it to the stir-fry right at the end to bring in more flavors and cook quickly.

Dinner: Curried chicken over cauliflower rice. Instead of serving this dish with regular rice, the cauliflower rice offers the added nutrient benefits of the vegetable while also providing a filling base for the meal. The curried flavors mixed into the lentils and chicken brings the dish alive.

Snack: Plain yogurt mixed with cinnamon and topped with fresh fruit. The yogurt offers a good source of protein, gut support, and additional anti-inflammatory benefits. The cinnamon is a good flavoring that works double to help you fight off inflammation. You can choose whatever fruit you want to top your yogurt with, but berries give a little extra anti-inflammatory boost to your snack.

Day 9:

Breakfast: Whole-grain oatmeal cooked in milk topped with fruits and a dollop of vanilla Greek yogurt. Choose a variety of fruits according to what is in season and your taste preference; however, choosing darker fruits offer the most anti-inflammatory properties.

Lunch: Tuna salad with a Mediterranean twist. Get a good serving of omega-3 fatty acid with a serving of tuna fish. You can serve your tuna salad over a mix of greens or on a piece of whole-grain toast. If you want to cut down on the salt of this recipe, put in fewer olives or capers and select a can of low-sodium tuna.

Dinner: Sautéed green beans served alongside mashed cannellini beans and a piece of grilled, high-quality steak. Make sure that your steak is trimmed and high quality. Remember, red meat should be a rare treat in your diet, so enjoy it when you serve it!

Snack: Fresh fruit, either one-cup of berries or a piece of stone fruit.

Day 10:

Breakfast: Green Goodness smoothie. Another smoothie option is a green smoothie, packed full of green fruits and vegetables. Try to get at least two servings of vegetables to one serving of fruit in this smoothie to offer the most nutrients in one cup.

Lunch: Mixed vegetable and lentil stew. The colors and flavors of this dish are hearty and delicious. Mix up the color lentil and the variety of vegetables if you want to change it up a little bit.

Dinner: Herbed, lemon zucchini, and salmon. When you steam your fish, you maintain all the flavor and moisture as well as all the nutrients. When you plate the vegetables and fish, pour a little of the liquid from the steamer onto the dish to add more flavor to the plate.

Snack: Fresh fruit, either one-cup of berries or a piece of stone fruit.

Day 11:

Breakfast: Vanilla Greek yogurt topped with organic granola or homemade granola with a variety of nuts, seeds, and oats. Sprinkle a few slices of fresh fruit or berries on top for extra flavor and anti-inflammatory benefits if you prefer.

Lunch: Tabbouleh with falafel. This true Mediterranean dish brings lentils to the forefront in a tasty little patty. If you want some additional protein, add grilled chicken or steamed fish, if you prefer.

Dinner: Rosemary and pecan topped tilapia. Selenium in tilapia is a good anti-inflammatory agent. In addition, this recipe is quick and easy but is decadent enough for a fancy dinner. The breadcrumbs can be replaced with a gluten-free version r almond flour if you prefer. Also, if you do not like the flavor of tilapia, swap this fish out for another option like cod or trout.

Snack: Slices of vegetables to dip into guacamole or hummus.

Day 12:

Breakfast: Ginger oatmeal. The amazing benefit of this dish is that it offers about ½ of your daily omega-3 fatty acid requirement without having to eat fish! It also packs a lot of flavors, almost like eating a piece of gingerbread.

Lunch: Sweet potato and roasted red pepper creamy soup. If you are looking to stock your freezer with meals to eat quickly, this is a recipe you should always have on hand. Roasting the vegetables prior to cooking them in the soup enhances the flavors. You can purchase pre-roasted red peppers in a jar, but to cut back on the sodium in the soup, consider roasting your own.

Dinner: "Burgers" made from black beans and sweet potatoes and served on bibb lettuce leaves. Dress your burger with toppings like sliced tomatoes, avocado, and red onion. Sprinkle a few sprouts on the top for extra help for your digestion. The sweet potato added to the "burger" mix brings beta-carotene and vitamin C that supports your health and fights back inflammation.

Snack: Plain yogurt mixed with cinnamon and topped with fresh fruit. The yogurt offers a good source of protein, gut support, and additional anti-inflammatory benefits. The cinnamon is a good flavoring that works double to help you fight off inflammation. You can choose whatever fruit you want to top your yogurt with, but berries give a little extra anti-inflammatory boost to your snack.

Day 13:

Breakfast: Frittata made with mushrooms and spinach. Like any egg dish, the flavors and combination of ingredients are practically endless. Mushrooms and spinach offer a good source of nutrients and flavor, but you can experiment with other vegetables according to your taste preference and what is available.

Lunch: Brown rice wrap filled with grilled chicken, chopped kale, shredded Parmesan cheese, and Caesar dressing. The brown rice wrap has the added benefit of being gluten-free, but the main objective is to offer a whole grain serving with your lunch. The kale offers a healthy backdrop to the chicken Caesar with it.Consider purchasing a pre-roasted chicken to make this even easier.

Dinner: Snapper and spinach served with a side of herbs and rice. Snapper is a good fish to get a serving of omega-3 fatty acids that you need for fighting inflammation. The spinach offers a good source of anti-inflammatory benefits, too. Served with the side of whole grain rice helps keep you full,and the fresh herbs add a nice aroma and flavor.

Snack: One cup of mixed, raw seeds and nuts

Day 14:

Breakfast: Vanilla Greek yogurt or coconut milk mixed with ginger and whole grain granola. The great thing about making your own granola is that you can make sure the ingredients are anti-inflammatory tasty.

Lunch: Curried squash and lentil stew. Another good soup to make early and either freeze or hold on to for another day. If you freeze it in lunch portions, you can just grab a container and go, letting it thaw throughout your morning. By lunchtime, it should be ready to eat!

Dinner: Basil and mozzarella pizza on a cauliflower crust. Spreading the crust with a light layer of fresh tomato sauce and then layering buffalo mozzarella and fresh basil leaves offer a healthy twist on a favorite "junk" food.

Snack: Slices of vegetables to dip into guacamole or hummus.

Day 15:

Breakfast: Porridge topped with dehydrated cherries. Whole grain oats or porridge sprinkled on top with dehydrated cherries provides a good serving of the antioxidant anthocyanin.

Lunch: Pumpkin soup. Pumpkin provides a lot of anti-inflammatory support in the form of beta-cryptoxanthin. To properly absorb this agent, you need the healthy fats found in this recipe. Make sure you select a high-quality source of pumpkin with strong skins. Cooking the soup with skins on makes this recipe even easier for you!

Dinner: Poached egg and curry potatoes with a side salad and vinaigrette.This is a simple dinner that you can make over and over. It is sure to fill you up and help you fight off inflammation. If poached eggs are not in your skill set or you do not like the taste, try cooking them in a skillet or boiling them to slice over the potatoes. Remember, eggs should come from a sustainable farm,and the chickens that they come from should be free-range. This makes sure you have the best serving of anti-inflammatory omega-3 fatty acids.

Snack: Mixed salad greens drizzled with extra virgin olive oil and balsamic vinegar. Choose high-quality vinegar to add to your salad. Not only will this enhance the taste but also you will get more benefits from this ingredient when chosen for quality over price.

Recipes

Breakfast:

Ginger and Whole-grain Granola

5 minutes prep, 45 minutes cook time

Ingredients:

Whole grain oats	2 cups
Buckwheat	1 cup
Sunflower seeds	1 cup
Pumpkin seeds	1 cup
Dates pitted	1 ½ cups
Apple sauce	1 cup
Coconut oil	6 Tbsp
Cocoa powder, raw, unsweetened	4 Tbsp
Ginger	1 nub

Directions:

1. Preheat your oven to 375 degrees Fahrenheit.
2. In a big bowl, toss the two types of seeds, buckwheat, and oats together until mixed well.
3. In a large pot, stir the applesauce, dates, and coconut oil together. Bring to a simmer over medium-low heat. Cook for about five minutes; make sure the dates are softened.
4. While the pot is simmering, peel and grate the ginger. Add it to the pot with the applesauce and dates.

5. Transfer the pot contents into a blender and add the cocoa to the container. Blend on high until the mixture is creamy.

6. Transfer the blender contents into the big mixing bowl full of seeds and oats. Stir well until all dry ingredients are coated.

7. Oil two large baking sheets with coconut oil and evenly spread the granola between the two pans.

8. Place the trays in the warmed oven and bake for 15 minutes. Remove trays from the oven and stir ingredients. Return the trays to the oven and cook five to ten minutes before removing the trays and stirring again. Do this for approximately 45 minutes or until the granola is crisp but not burnt. This process ensures that all the ingredients are evenly toasted and browned.

9. When the granola is done the cooking, place the trays on the counter to cool completely. Once room temperature, transfer the contents into a container that has an airtight seal. It will keep for about one month.

Easy Crepes

7 minutes prep, 3 minutes cook time. Makes about six crepes.

Ingredients:

Eggs	2 medium
Vanilla extract	1 Tsp
Almond milk	½ cup
Water	½ cup
Salt	¼ tsp
Agave nectar	2 Tbsp
Gluten-free all-purpose flour	1 cup
Melted coconut oil	2 Tbsp + 1 Tbsp for greasing pan

Directions:

1. Over low heat, in a little saucepan, melt the 2 Tbsp of coconut oil.
2. Whisk the agave, water, milk, vanilla, and eggs in a medium-sized bowl.
3. Begin adding the flour to the wet ingredients a little at a time, whisking in between additions.
4. Pour the melted coconut oil into the batter, slowly and continuously, then whisk well.
5. Place a larger frying pan over medium-high heat and use the remaining 1 Tbsp of coconut oil to grease the bottom of the pan.
6. Pour about 1/3 cup of the batter into the pan and swirl

the batter around the pan by tilting the pan in a circle,so the batter reaches the edges of the pan and is evenly distributed.

7. Cook about 2 minutes on this side, lightly browning the bottom. Flip over and cook about another minute on the other side.

8. Continue until all the batter is used.

Morning Muffins Made with Ginger, Apple, and Rhubarb

15 minutes prep, 25 minutes cook time. Makes about eight muffins.

Ingredients:

Almond flour	½ cup
Sugar, unrefined, raw	¼ cup
Crystallized ginger, chopped	2 Tbsp
Ground flaxseed	1 Tbsp
Buckwheat flour	½ cup
Brown rice flour, fine	¼ cup
Arrowroot powder	2 Tbsp
Baking powder, gluten-free	2 tsp
Cinnamon, ground	½ tsp
Ginger, ground	½ tsp
Sea salt	Pinch
Rhubarb, sliced	1 cup
Apple, cored, peeled, diced	1 small
Extra virgin olive oil	¼ cup
Almond milk	1/3 cup + 1 Tbsp
Egg	1 large
Vanilla extract	1 tsp

Directions:

1. Preheat your oven to 350 degrees Fahrenheit. Prepare a muffin tin with liners or grease the cups well.
2. In a medium-sized mixing bowl, combine the ground flaxseed, ginger, sugar, and almond flour.
3. Using a fine sieve, sift the flours and powder into the bowl. Do the same for the cinnamon and ground ginger. Whisk together.
4. Mix in the apple dices and slices of rhubarb into the flour mixture and toss to coat evenly.
5. In a small-sized mixing bowl, combine the vanilla, egg, oil, and milk and whisk well. Transfer the wet ingredients to the dry bowl and stir to combine.
6. Spoon the mixture into the muffin tins, filling each cup about ¾ full for the best results. Tops with diced apple or sliced rhubarb, if you prefer and have extra on hand.
7. Place the muffin tin into the oven and cook for about 20 minutes, or until a toothpick comes out clean when inserted into the middle of a muffin.
8. Remove the tin from the oven when done baking and allow to cool for five minutes before eating. Store in a container with an airtight lid for up to three days.

Lunch:

Potato and Smoked Salmon Tartine

25 minutes prep, 20 minutes cook time. Makes one tartine, serves about two.

Ingredients:

Potato, russet, peeled, grated	1 large
Extra virgin olive oil	2 Tbsp
Salt and pepper	Dash
Goat cheese, room temperature	4 Ozs
Chives, minced	1 ½ Tbsp. + more for topping
Garlic, minced	½ clove
Salmon, smoked	As desired, about 8 Oz.
Lemon, zest	½ medium
Capers, drained	2 Tbsp.
Red onion, diced	2 Tbsp.
Egg, hard-boiled, chopped	½ medium

Directions:

1. In a small mixing bowl, stir the garlic, lemon zest, and goat cheese until combined. Add salt and pepper as desired. Fold in 1½ Tbsp. chives and place the bowl to the side.

2. In another small bowl, add the red onion and egg. Season with salt and pepper as desired. Set this bowl aside as well.

3. Warm the olive oil in a large frying pan over medium-high heat.

4. Quickly shred the potato into a cheesecloth and wring out the potatoes over the sink to remove the extra liquid from the potatoes. Season with salt and pepper as desired and gently mix to combine.

5. Add the potato to the hot pan and spread out with a spoon into a circular shape. Press down the potatoes to bring the pieces together. Place a lid over the pan and cook for about ten minutes. The bottom should be a light brown color.

6. Using a spatula, flip the tartine over to cook on the other side, approximately another ten minutes.

7. Transfer the potato tartine from the pan to a cooling rack and let it cool to the temperature of the room.

8. Once cool, use a spoon or knife to spread the goat cheese mixture over the potatoes. Then add the smoked salmon to the top of the goat cheese. Add the red onion and egg mixture over the salmon and top with the capers. Sprinkle the remaining chives on top and cut like a pizza to serve.

Sweet Potato and Roasted Red Pepper Creamy Soup

25 minutes prep, 30 minutes cook time. Makes about six servings.

Ingredients:

Extra virgin olive oil	2 Tbsp.
Onion, chopped	2 medium
Roasted red peppers, chopped, reserved liquid	12 Oz.
Green chili, diced	4 Oz.
Cumin, ground	2 tsp.
Salt	1 tsp.
Coriander, ground	1 tsp.
Sweet potatoes, peeled, cubed	4 cups
Vegetable or bone broth	4 cups
Cilantro, minced	2 Tbsp.
Lemon juice	1 Tbsp.
Cream cheese, cubed	4 oz.

Directions:

1. Warm the olive oil in a large soup pot over medium-high heat.
2. When hot, place the onion inside and heat until softened.
3. Mix in the coriander, salt, cumin, chilis, and red peppers and stir often for about 2 minutes.
4. Pour in the reserved liquid from the red peppers and then add the broth and sweet potatoes. Boil and then lower to a simmer, placing a lid on top to cook for about 15

minutes.

5. After 15 minutes, remove the lid and stir the lemon juice and cilantro into the mixture. Allow cooling for a few minutes.

6. Pour the soup into the blender and add the cream cheese. Pulse the soup until creamy. Pour back into the pot to warm again. Add more salt if desired.

Tuna Salad with a Mediterranean Twist

3 minutes prep, 12 minutes cook time. Makes about two servings.

Ingredients:

Water-packed tuna, drained	2 5-ounce cans
Mayonnaise	¼ cup
Olives, chopped	¼ cup
Red onion, minced	2 Tbsp.
Red peppers, roasted, chopped	2 Tbsp.
Basil, chopped	2 Tbsp.
Capers	1 Tbsp.
Lemon juice	1 Tbsp.
Salt and pepper	Dash
Tomatoes, optional	2 large

Directions:

1. In a large mixing bowl, add the lemon juice, capers, basil, red peppers, onion, olives, mayonnaise, and tuna fish. Season with salt and pepper as desired. Mix well.

2. Slice open the tomatoes into six pieces but do not cut all the way through. Scoop the tuna salad into the inside of the tomatoes. If you do not want to serve in a tomato, consider adding it to the top of mixed greens or with whole grain crackers for a dip.

Dinner:

Poached Egg and Curry Potatoes

10 minutes prep, 30 minutes cook time. Makes about four servings.

Ingredients:

Potato, russet, cubed	2 large
Ginger, peeled, minced	1 in. nub
Garlic, minced	2 cloves
Extra virgin olive oil	1 Tbsp.
Curry powder	2 Tbsp.
Tomato sauce	15 oz.
Eggs	4 large
Cilantro, chopped	½ bunch

Directions:

1. Warm water in a large stockpot and add the potatoes. Cover and boil on high heat for about five minutes. Drain and set aside.
2. Warm the oil in a large skillet over medium-low heat. Ass the garlic and ginger and cook for about two minutes. Stir

in the curry powder and cook for another minute.

3. Pour in the tomato sauce into the skillet and mix well. Increase the heat to medium and warm. Add salt if desired.

4. Carefully add the potatoes, taking care not to splash the sauce. Mix to cover the potatoes. Add a bit of water to the skillet if the sauce is too thick.

5. Push the sauce and potatoes aside, creating four wells to add the eggs. Crack each egg into the skillet. Cover and cook for about ten minutes or until eggs are well-cooked. Sprinkle cilantro on top, if desired.

Turkey Chili

10 minutes prep, six hours cook time. Makes about ten servings.

Ingredients:

Extra virgin olive oil	1 Tbsp.
Onion, diced	1 medium
Turkey, ground	1 lb.
Red pepper, chopped	1 medium
Yellow pepper, chopped	1 medium
Tomato sauce	2 15-ounce cans
Tomatoes, petite diced	2 15-ounce cans
Black beans, drained, rinsed	2 15-ounce cans
Red kidney beans, drained, rinsed	2 15-ounce cans
Jalapeno peppers, jarred, sliced, drained	16 oz.
Chili powder	2 Tbsp.

Cumin, ground	1 Tbsp.
Salt and pepper	Dash

Directions:

1. Warm the olive oil in a large pan over medium-high heat. Add the turkey when the pan is hot and brown. Add it to your slow cooker.
2. Top the turkey with the remaining ingredients.
3. Set your slow cooker on low and cook the chili for about six hours.

Red Bell Peppers Stuffed with Italian Filling

10 minutes prep, 30 minutes cook time. Makes about four servings.

Ingredients:

Potato, russet, cubed	2 large

Directions:

1. Warm your oven to 450 degrees Fahrenheit. Prepare a baking tray with tin foil and an oil rub to prevent sticking.
2. Wash the red peppers and remove the stem and seeds. Cut in half.
3. Warm the olive oil in a large skillet over medium heat. Add the turkey and cook until browned. Before full cooked, stir in the sauce and herbs to the skillet. Continue

to stir while cooking for about four more minutes or until no longer pink.

4. Stir in the parmesan cheese and spinach until fully mixed in.

5. Place ½ cup of the turkey mixture into the halves of peppers and top each with one tablespoon of grated parmesan cheese.

6. Place the tray into the oven and cook for about 30 minutes or until the cheese is browned slightly and melted.

"Burgers" Made from Black Beans and Sweet Potatoes

Up to 50 minutes prep, 30 minutes for setting, 8 minutes cook time. Makes about six servings.

Ingredients:

Quinoa, cooked	1 ½ cup
Black beans, drained, rinsed	1 15-ounce can
Sweet potato, peeled, cubed	1 large
Red onion, diced	½ cup
Garlic, minced	2 cloves
Cilantro, chopped	½ cup + 2 Tbsp. for cream
Jalapeno, diced, seed removed	½ medium
Cumin, ground	1 tsp.
Cajun seasoning	2 tsp.
Oat Flour	¼ cup
Salt and pepper	Dash
Extra virgin olive oil	As needed
Sprouts	As desired

Bib lettuce	6 leaves
Avocado, diced	½ large
Greek yogurt, plain	¼ cup
Lime juice	1 tsp.
Hot sauce, optional	Dash
Salt	Dash

Directions:

1. Cook the sweet potatoes for about four minutes or until soft. If roasting the potatoes, place them on a baking tray in an oven pre-heated to 400 degrees Fahrenheit. Roast them for about 30 minutes. Remove the skins when cooked.

2. Place the sweet potatoes into a blender. Add the black beans, Cajun seasoning, cumin, garlic, cilantro, and red onion and blend until smooth.

3. In a large mixing bowl, transfer the blender ingredients in with the cooked quinoa. Stir together until combined. Season with salt and pepper if desired.

4. Stir in the flour to thicken the mixture. You may not need the entire amount.

5. Form the mixture into six "burgers," using about ½ cup of the mixture for each patty. Place on parchment paper and cool them in the fridge for about 30 minutes.

6. While cooling, make the avocado cream. In the blender or food processor, add the avocado, lime juice, and remaining cilantro. Pulse until creamy. Add to the fridge

to cool with the patties.

7. When ready to cook, warm olive oil in a large skillet over medium-high heat. Place the "burgers" into the skillet and cook for about four minutes on each side. Serve with the cream on top when done.

Red Bell Peppers Stuffed with Quinoa and Ground Turkey

10 minutes prep, 35 minutes cook time. Makes about six servings.

Ingredients:

Red bell peppers	3 large
Turkey, ground	1 ¼ lb.
Mushrooms, diced	1 cup
Sweet onion, diced	¼ cup
Spinach, chopped	1 cup
Tomato sauce	1 cup
Vegetable or bone broth	1 cup
Quinoa, cooked	2 cups

Directions:

1. In a medium skillet, warm the oil and sauté the vegetables for about five minutes over medium heat.

2. Stir in the turkey and garlic, cooking until almost cooked through.

3. Pour in the tomato sauce and ½ cup of broth into the skillet. Simmer until the turkey is fully cooked and some

of the liquid has cooked off.

4. While the turkey is cooking, warm your oven to 400 degrees Fahrenheit. Prepare the bell peppers by removing the stems, cutting in half, and removing the seeds. Prepare the baking dish with tin foil and a coating of oil to prevent sticking.

5. Stir in the quinoa into the pan with the turkey and stir to combine. When the turkey is fully cooked, scoop the mixture into the peppers, about ½ cup per pepper. Place the peppers into the baking dish. Pour the remaining ½ cup of broth around the peppers.

6. Cover the baking dish with tin foil and place in the oven. Cook for about 35 minutes.

Chapter 7: Conversation Tables

When you sit around the table and explain to someone that you are going to be adopting the anti-inflammatory lifestyle, you may be met with some blank stares or a host of other opinions of how you should take charge of your health. No matter what you encounter, it is best to be prepared for how you will discuss your new diet and lifestyle in a way that is accessible, accepting, and appropriate. The purpose of this chapter is to give you some conversational guides to navigate from the naïve to the nasty.

It is time to alter the conversation surrounding the concept of "total" or "whole" care. This means taking a proactive approach to your well-being that is customized to your own needs. It is also an approach that requires ownership over your medical care, beyond just being driven by a medical professional. You are responsible for learning and responding to your body's needs, not relying on a doctor or medical professional to interpret your symptoms when they have gone too far. And part of this process of mixing professional and self-care includes having a supportive community. This community is what will help keep you on track or derail you immediately. Having a series of go-to statements that can help educate your community to support your health initiatives is what changes your health goals from wishes to reality. It is what moves the needle from good, focused care to well-rounded total health.

Introducing What Inflammation Is

1. A natural process for protection that your body uses to fight off infections and injuries.
2. Compare inflammation to fire; in small and controlled situations it is good and warm, but if it spreads uncontrollably it can cause a catastrophe.
3. Inflammation can become the disease if it is out of control in your body.
4. Serious medical conditions are linked to chronic, or out of control, inflammation in the body, such as asthma, cancer, fibromyalgia, and heart disease.

Food and Inflammation

1. There are many theories about how food and inflammation interact with one another, which is partly why we know a lot about physical reactions to foods within your body but also why there is still controversy surrounding the diet.
   a. One Theory: Eicosanoids are the product of broken-down omega-3 and omega-6 fatty acids. These molecules tell and control the body in relation to your immune system and inflammation. They also transport messages back

and forth from the central nervous system. If you eat too much omega-6 fatty acids, you are signaling more inflammation to occur in your body, but omega-3 fatty acids signal anti-inflammation. Omega-6 is found in meats, fats, and preservatives. Omega-3 is found in oily fish.

b. Second Theory: Your gut's microbiome contains bacterial flora that helps your general health when it is healthy, but when it is out of balance it can allow unhealthy bacteria to grow, causing poor health and various illnesses. Income extreme cases doctors will transplant another person's fecal matter into your gut to balance your bacteria because your gut can no longer self-adjust from your diet. Currently, there is much study underway to determine the exact kinds of bacteria that should grow in your gut and at what levels to determine optimal health.

c. Third Theory: Free radicals are closely tied to the level of inflammation in your body at any given time. These little compounds offer different chemical reactions their electrons in order to ward off infection. But it has been found that excessive levels of free radicals in the body can aggravate inflammation and damage your tissue.

Supplements can be prescribed to help regulate the levels of free radicals using antioxidants, but the benefits and safety of these additives are uncertain. Most doctors recommend fighting free radicals by consuming foods rich in antioxidants.

The Science Behind the Diet

1. Researchers have found several diseases that are connected to increased levels of inflammation in your body. These include:

   a. Autoimmune disease- Scleroderm, and arthritis are examples of illnesses when the body begins to attack itself. Eating a vegetarian diet and increasing the oil from fish have been shown to help alleviate some of the pain associated with these conditions.

   b. Asthma- The people that eat a large amount of fast food tend to have poorly-controlled asthma. Eating more fish oil can help reduce medication dependency and help your airway stay open, especially if asthma symptoms worsen from exercise.

   c. Alzheimer's disease- Your memory is at risk when you eat a diet that is high in carbohydrates. To help protect your mind, you should consume a moderate amount of red wine, whole grain cereal, and oily fish's omega-3 fatty acids. Even monounsaturated fats have been shown to help protect your mind.

d. Chronic lung diseases, such as bronchitis and emphysema- Oxygen can be increased in the bloodstream by eating more omega-3 fatty acids. In addition, more omega-3's can help dyspnea and reduce cytokines, known for causing inflammation.

e. Cancers- Of all the cancer diagnosis in the United States, about 35% is connected to a poor diet. To help prevent cancer it has been found that a diet rich in vegetables and fruits that are high in antioxidants is recommended.

f. Fibromyalgia or chronic pain disorders- There is a small study published linking a vegan diet to pain dissolution. Another study showed that an anti-inflammatory diet could help alleviate pain and reduce possibly painful enzymes, such as phospholipase-A2.

g. Heart disease- A large study on over 10,000 participants showed that an anti-inflammatory diet helped reduce the risk of heart disease in half!

h. Inflammatory bowel disease, ulcerative colitis, or Crohn's disease- In clinical trials, steroid use was significantly reduced when participants followed a diet rich in selenium, vitamin E, vitamin C, fructo-oligosaccharides, and fish oil.

i. Type-2 diabetes- Chronic inflammation is found in nearly all people diagnosed with type-2 diabetes. It is therefore recommended to those that are pre-diabetic, or at risk of developing diabetes, to follow an anti-inflammatory diet to mitigate the disease.

2. In a recent publication, a healthy diet has the ability to prevent nearly 60% of all chronic diseases.

3. Following an anti-inflammatory diet can help prevent and lower the risk of developing the illnesses presented earlier.

Foods and The Anti-Inflammatory Diet

1. Foods are encouraged and discouraged based on their link to their known connection to inflammation in the body.

2. Preserved foods, fast foods, and animal products tend to have omega-6 fatty acids, saturated fats, and trans fats, which are all known to encourage chronic inflammation.

3. Extra virgin olive oil, oily fish, fruits, and vegetables tend to have monounsaturated fats, omega-3 fatty acids, and DHA.

4. Extra virgin olive oil is a preferred cooking oil because research has shown its ability to reduce LDL levels, c-reactive proteins, fasting glucose, and systolic blood pressure. When heated it also resists conversion of trans fatty acid.

5. Vegetables and fruits that are dark in color, like deep green or dark blue, are typically rich in flavonoids, which are a signal for high nutritional content.

6. Avoiding juice is beneficial because it tends to have high levels of sugar and often additional sugars are added for flavor. Juice also strips the fiber out of the fruit or vegetable.

7. Fiber is essential to a healthy diet and can significantly decrease inflammation. CRP is negatively impacted when

you eat grains that have more than 23 grams of fiber. 30 grams per day is recommended.

8. Free radicals are formed most when insulin levels are high,and so are post-prandial glucose. These levels are raised after consumption of foods with an elevated glycemic load, such as carbohydrates that have been highly processed. The glycemic load of carbohydrate is the one best consideration for a potential inflammatory response.

9. Animal proteins tend to have a higher amount of unhealthy fats, which cause inflammation, so protein should be consumed in plant form as often as possible. These sources include soy-based options, nuts, grains, and legumes.

10. If you must eat animal protein, you should choose sustainably raised and grass-fed animal meat or wild-caught sources. Always trim off visible fat before and after cooking meats and do not "char" or burn the meat, as this can lead to additional inflammatory responses.

11. Fish are good sources of protein, but it is important to choose options that typically are less impacted by the high levels of mercury in the water. This means avoiding large fish like shark and bass, or fish that eat other fish as their primary diet. The best fish to consume include anchovies, salmon, and tilapia.

12. Beverages do not have to be limited to water only. It has been shown in clinical studies that a single glass of red wine has the ability to lower inflammation in the body. Up to six glasses of green tea can also help lower inflammation as well as the risk for developing cancer. You can add fresh fruit or vegetables to fruit for flavoring, but it should be as unaltered as possible most of the time.

13. Spices and herbs are the preferred methods for seasoning your food. Some flavorings are more anti-inflammatory than others, such as cayenne pepper, cumin, clove, rosemary, ginger, oregano, and turmeric. It is a good practice to have those on hand to add to a dish for flavor and anti-inflammation support.

14. For a sweet treat, eating a single ounce of dark chocolate can help lower inflammation and offer a nice evening treat. The chocolate should be more than 70% cocoa.

Some "Rules" of Empowered Eating for Your Health and Anti-inflammation

1. If your great-grandmother would not understand it as food, stay away from it.
2. If the food will "god bad" or compost one day, it is good to eat in its prime.
3. Check the ingredient label. If one of the top three ingredients is sugar, avoid it.
4. Try to make your plate full of natural color.
5. If the milk changes color when you put the cereal in it, do not eat it.
6. Pay attention to if you are full or getting close. Try to stop eating before you feel full.
7. Sit at the table to eat your meals, not on the couch, at a desk, in a bed, etc.
8. When choosing meat, go with the fewest feet. If it has two instead of four feet, it is a better choice. No feet are even better!
9. However long it took to cook your meal is how long you should spend enjoying it, at the very least.
10. Desserts are for special occasions; treat them that way.
11. It is ok to break the rules now and then!

Diet Versus Lifestyle Conversation

1. A diet is a single choice regarding what foods and drinks you consume. A lifestyle is a choice of how you want to live and includes decisions like how you sleep, move, and eat.

2. Supporting a healthy diet with other healthy choices enhances the health benefits of the foods and drinks you ingest and can bring the benefits faster.

3. Some additional lifestyle considerations that pair well with the anti-inflammatory diet include:

   a. Balancing your work and life

   b. Deal with daily stress in a healthy manner, such as through meditation or therapy.

   c. Be an active member of a community of like-minded people, meaning the people are also pursuing actions and choices that support their health and well-being.

   d. In addition to being in a community of those also focused on their health, choose to be around people that love and support you.

   e. Get outside in the fresh air and sunshine as often as possible.

   f. Be physically active at least 20 minutes every day. This can be in a combination of five minutes at a time adding up to 20 minutes, and it does not have to be "exercising," but rather walking for a few minutes or taking the stairs when possible.

g. Get at least seven hours of quality sleep a night. Develop an evening routine that supports a positive sleeping habit to give your body time to rest and renew.

The Case Against Non-Steroidal Anti-inflammatory Drugs, or NSAID's

1. Many diseases are being treated with NSAID's, such as arthritis and even heart diseases, to help lower inflammation in the body but long-term side effects can be dangerous.

2. Recent studies have shown that long-term treatment with NSAID's lead to heart problems, such as myocardial infection or ischemic heart failure, and are life-threatening.

3. NSAID's work by inhibiting certain enzymes so your body lowers inflammation without causing stomach discomfort or bowel interference, but prolonging the use of the medications can be more dangerous than helpful.

4. Some of the negative side effects of NSAID's include:

   a. Stomach ulcers- if you are prone to ulcers, NSAID's should be taken only under medical supervision and sparingly. These can not only be painful but dangerous to your health.

   b. Stomach discomfort- this is a mild side effect and occurs most often in those that tend to develop GI issues or upsets.

c. Hypertension- this is a common side effect for those that use NSAID's for an extended period. It often leads to the next side effect.

d. Stroke- this is another common side effect for long-term use. If serious enough it can cause incapacitation or death.

e. Increased bleeding risk- NSAID's can thin your blood, making wounds bleed more than usual. Sometimes this is mild or easily remedied; however, for others and those needing surgery, it can be more bothersome.

f. Issues with your kidneys- certain NSAID's are processed through the kidneys,and it can be very hard on the organ. If you suffer from other kidney problems, it may be advisable to not take NSAID's, even in the short-term.

5. To offset the negative side effects or treat these inflammatory diseases, natural remedies are recommended.

6. Some of the natural products being considered include curcumin, zedoarondiol, a-cyperone, kaurenoic acid, and berberine.

a. Curcumin- a derivative from turmeric

b. Zedoarondiol- a derivative from turmeric

c. A-cyperone- isolated from nutgrass

d. Kaurenoic acid - isolated from the croton antisyphilitics Mart plant or weed

e. Berberine- extracted from a variety of plant sources, including berberis, goldenseal, and barberry

7. Additional treatment for various inflammatory issues includes resting the body as often as possible, especially if battling an inflammatory disease or response. If an area is swollen, applying ice and compression also seem to help relieve symptoms. If possible, you can elevate the area above your heart and head, which can also help reduce swelling and inflammation.

References

Scientific Journal Resources:

1. Adam O, Beringer C, Kless T, et al. "Anti-Inflammatory Effects Of A Low Arachidonic Acid Diet And Fish Oil In Patients With Rheumatoid Arthritis." Rheumatol Institute. 2003; 23(1): 27-36.
2. Anand P, Kunnumakara AB, Sundaram C, et al. "Cancer Is A Preventable Disease That Requires Major Lifestyle Changes." Pharmaceutical Resource. 2008; 25(9): 2097-2116.
3. Barzi F, Woodward M, Marfisi R, Tavazzi L, Valagussa F, Marchioli R. "Mediterranean Diet And All-Causes Mortality After Myocardial Infarction: Results From The GISSI-Prevenzione Trial." European Journal of Clinical Nutrition. 2003; 57(4): 604-611.
4. Bergmans RS, Palta M, Robert SA, Berger LM, Ehrenthal DB, Malecki KM. "Associations Between Food Security Status and Dietary Inflammatory Potential within Lower-Income Adults from the United States National Health and Nutrition Examination Survey, Cycles2007 to 2014." Journal of Academic Nutrition and Diet. 2018; 118(6): 994- 1005.
5. Cha, R.J., Zeng, D.W., Chang, Q.S. "Non-Surgical Treatment Of Small Cell Lung Cancer With Chemo-Radio-Immunotherapy And Traditional Chinese Medicine." ZhonghuaNeiKe Za Zhi. 1994; 33: 462–466.
6. Chen, L., Xie, C., Wu, L. "Point Injection Of Radici Astragali For Treatment Of Post-Chemotherapy Adverse Reactions." Journal of Traditional Chinese Medicine. 2005; 25: 21–22.
7. Chen, X.J., Bian, Z.P., Lu, S., Xu, J.D., Gu, C.R., Yang, D., Zhang, J.N. "Cardiac Protective Effect Of *Astragalus* On Viral Myocarditis Mice: Comparison With Perindopril."

The American Journal of Chinese Medicine. 2006; 34: 493–502.

8. Chi, H., Barry, S.P., Roth, R.J., Wu, J.J., Jones, E.A., Bennett, A.M., Flavell, R.A., 2006. Dynamic regulation of pro- and anti-inflammatory cytokines by MAPK phosphatase 1 (MKP-1) in innate immune responses. Proceedings of the National Academy of Sciences of the United States of America 103, 2274–2279.

9. Chow, C.C., Clermont, G., Kumar, R., Lagoa, C., Tawadrous, Z., Gallo, D., Betten, B., Bartels, J., Constantine, G., Fink, M.P., Billiar, T.R., Vodovotz, Y. "The Acute Inflammatory Response In Diverse Shock States." Shock. 2005; 24: 74–84.

10. Chu, D.T., Lepe-Zuniga, J., Wong, W.L., LaPushin, R., Mavligit, G.M., 1988. Fractional extract of *Astragalus membranaceus*, a Chinese medicinal herb, potentiates LAK cell cytotoxicity generated by a low dose of recombinant interleukin-2. Journal of Clinical and Laboratory Immunology 26, 183–187.

11. Craig WJ. "Phytochemicals: Guardians Of Our Health." Journal of American Diet Association. 1997; 97(10): S199-S204.

12. Cross, A.S., Opal, S.M. "A New Paradigm For The Treatment Of Sepsis: Is It Time To Consider Combination Therapy?" Annotated Journal of Internal Medicine; 138: 502–505.

13. D'Andrea, A., ste-Amezaga, M., Valiante, N.M., Ma, X., Kubin, M., Trinchieri, G. "Interleukin 10 (IL-10) Inhibits Human Lymphocyte Interferon Gamma-Production By Suppressing Natural Killer Cell Stimulatory Factor/IL-12 Synthesis In Accessory Cells." Journal of Experimental Medicine. 1993; 178: 1041–1048.

14. Day, J., Rubin, J., Vodovotz, Y., Chow, C.C., Reynolds, A., Clermont, G. "A Reduced Mathematical Model Of The Acute Inflammatory Response II. Capturing Scenarios Of Repeated Endotoxin Administration." Journal of Theoretical Biology, in press. 2006.

15. *"Diet Wars II: How Do The Plans Measure Up?"* Harvard Men's Health Watch. 2003; 7(6): 1-5.
16. Doll R, Peto R. "The Causes Of Cancer: Quantitative Estimates Of Avoidable Risks Of Cancer In The United States Today." Journal of National Cancer Institute. 1981; 66(6): 1192-1308.
17. Dong, C., Davis, R.J., Flavell, R.A., 2002. "MAP kinases in the immune response." Annual Review of Immunology 20, 55–72.
18. Estruch R, Martínez-González MA, Corella D, et al. "Effects Of A Mediterranean-Style Diet On Cardiovascular Risk Factors: A Randomized Trial." Annotated International Journal of Medicine. 2006; 145(1): 1-11.
19. Farhangi MA, Najafi M. "Dietary Inflammatory Index: A Potent Association With Cardiovascular Risk Factors Among Patients Candidate For Coronary Artery Bypass Grafting (CABG) Surgery." Nutritional Journal. 2018; 17(1):20.
20. Fuchs, A.C., Granowitz, E.V., Shapiro, L., Vannier, E., Lonnemann, G., Angel, J.B., Kennedy, J.S., Rabson, A.R., Radwanski, E., Affrime, M.B., Cutler, D.L., Grint, P.C., Dinarello, C.A. "Clinical, Hematologic, And Immunologic Effects Of Interleukin-10 In Humans." Journal of Clinical Immunology. 1996; 16: 291–303.
21. Furst, R., Schroeder, T., Eilken, H.M., Bubik, M.F., Kiemer, A.K., Zahler, S., Vollmar, A.M., 2007. "MAPK phosphatase-1 represents a noveanti-inflammatory target of glucocorticoids in the human endothelium." The FASEB Journal 21, 74–80.
22. Giugliano D, Esposito K. "Mediterrananean Diet and Metabolic Diseases." Current Opinion Lipidol. 2008; 19(1): 63-68.
23. Hei, Z.Q., Huang, H.Q., Zhang, J.J., Chen, B.X., Li, X.Y., 2005. "Protective effect of *Astragalus membranaceus*on intestinal mucosa reperfusion injury after hemorrhagic shock in rats." World Journal of Gastroenterology 11, 4986–4991.

24. Henderson ST. "High Carbohydrate Diets And Alzheimer's Disease. Medical Hypotheses."2004; 62(5): 689-700.
25. Ji, L.L., Gomez-Cabrera, M.C., Vina, J., 2006. "Exercise and hormesis: activation of cellular antioxidant signaling pathway." Annals of the New York Academy Sciences 1067, 425–435.
26. Jin, R., Wan, L.L., Mitsuishi, T., Kodama, K., Kurashige, S., 1994. "Immunomodulative effects of Chinese herbs in mice treated with anti-tumor agent cyclophosphamide." YakugakuZasshi: Journal of the Pharmaceutical Society of Japan 114, 533–538.
27. Jung, C.H., Kim, J.H., Hong, M.H., Seog, H.M., Oh, S.H., Lee, P.J., Kim, G.J., Kim, H.M., Um, J.Y., Ko, S.-G., 2007. "Phenolic-rich fraction from *Rhusvernicifllua*Stokes (RVS) suppress inflammatory response via NF-B and JNK pathway in LPS-induced RAW 264.7 macrophages." Journal of Ethnopharmacology 110, 490–497.
28. Kapka-Skrzypczak L, Niedźwiecka J, Skrzypczak M, Kruszewski M. "Nutrients As Inflammatory State Modulators." Pediatric Endocrinal Diabetes Metabolism. 2013; 19(1): 39-43.
29. Kohatsu W. "The Anti-Inflammatory Diet." Integrative Medicine. 3rd ed. Philadelphia, PA: Saunders, WH; 2010.
30. Kontogianni MD, Zampelas A, Tsigos C. "Nutrition and Inflammation Load." Academic Science. 2006; 1083 (214): 38.
31. Kumar, R., Clermont, G., Vodovotz, Y., Chow, C.C. "The Dynamics Of Acute Inflammation." Journal of TheoreticaBiologygy. 2004; 230: 145–155.
32. Kusum, M., Klinbuayaem, V., Bunjob, M., Sangkitporn, S., 2004. "Preliminary efficacy and safety of oral suspension SH, combination of five Chinese medicinal herbs, in people living with HIV/AIDS; the phase I/II study." Journal of the Medical Association of Thailand 87, 1065–1070.
33. Lee, Y.S., Han, O.K., Park, C.W., Yang, C.H., Jeon, T.W., Yoo, W.K., Kim, S.H., Kim, H.J., 2005. "Pro-

inflammatory cytokine gene expression and nitric oxide regulation of aqueous extracted Astragali radix in Raw 264.7 macrophage cells." Journal of Ethnopharmacology 100, 289–294.

34. Li D, Ng A, Mann NJ, Sinclair AJ. "Contribution Of Meat Fat To Dietary Arachidonic Acid." Lipids. 1998; 33(4): 437-440.

35. Matsuyama W, Mitsuyama H, Watanabe M, et al. "Effects Of Omega-3 Polyunsaturated Fatty Acids On Inflammatory Markers In COPD." CHEST Journal. 2005; 128(6): 3817-3827.

36. Marshall, J.C., "Clinical Trials Of Mediator-Directed Therapy In Sepsis: What Have We Learned?" Intensive Care Medicine. 2000; 26 (Suppl. 1): 75–83.

37. Minihane, A. M., Vinoy, S., Russell, W. R., Baka, A., et al. (2015). "Low-grade inflammation, diet composition,and health: current research evidence and its translation." The British journal of nutrition, 2015; 114(7): 999-1012.

38. Nick, J.A., Coldren, C.D., Geraci, M.W., Poch, K.R., Fouty, B.W., O'Brien, J., Gruber, M., Zarini, S., Murphy, R.C., Kuhn, K., Richter, D., Kast, K.R., Abraham, E. "Recombinant Human Activated Protein C Reduces Human Endotoxin-Induced Pulmonary Inflammation Via Inhibition Of Neutrophil Chemotaxis." Blood. 2004; 104 (13): 3878–3885.

39. Panza F, Solfrizzi V, Colacicco A, et al. "Mediterranean Diet And Cognitive Decline." Public Health Nutrition. 2004; 7(07): 959-963.

40. Paulsen, F., Pufe, T., Conradi, L., Varoga, D., Tsokos, M., Papendieck, J., Petersen, W. "Antimicrobial Peptides Are Expressed And Produced In Healthy And Inflamed Human Synovial Membranes." Journal of Pathology. 2002; 198: 369–377.

41. Phillips CM, Shivappa N, Hébert JR, Perry IJ. "Dietary Inflammatory Index and Biomarkers of Lipoprotein Metabolism, Inflammation and Glucose Homeostasis in Adults." Nutrients. 2018; 10(8): E1033.

42. Rakel DP, Rindfleisch A. "Inflammation: Nutritional, Botanical, And Mind-Body Influences." Southern Medical Journal. 2005; 98(3): 303-310.
43. Ren Z, Zhao A, Wang Y, Meng L, Szeto IM, Li T, Gong H, Tian Z, Zhang Y, Wang P. "Association between Dietary Inflammatory Index, C-Reactive Protein and Metabolic Syndrome: A Cross-Sectional Study." Nutrients. 2018: 10(7): E831.
44. Schulze MB, Hoffmann K, Manson JE, et al. "Dietary Pattern, Inflammation, And Incidence Of Type 2 Diabetes In Women." American Journal of Clinical Nutrition. 2005; 82(3): 675-684.
45. Seaman DR. "The Diet-Induced Pro-Inflammatory State." Journal of Manipulative Physical Therapy. 2002; 25(3): 168-179.
46. Sears B. "Anti-inflammatory Diets for Obesity and Diabetes." Journal of American College of Nutrition. 2009; 28: 482S- 491S.
47. Stvrtinova, V., Jakubovsky, J., Hulin, I. "The Acute Phase Reactants." Inflammation and Fever. Academic Electronic Press. 1995.
48. Takala, A., Jousela, I., Jansson, S.E., Olkkola, K.T., Takkunen, O., Orpana, A., Karonen, S.L., Repo, H."Markers Of Systemic Inflammation Predicting Organ Failure In Community-Acquired Septic Shock." Clinical Science. (London) 1999; 97: 529–538.
49. Tracey, K.J. "High mobility group 1 protein (HMG-1) stimulateproinflammatorycytokine synthesis in human monocytes." Journal of Experimental Medicine. 2000; 192: 565–570.
50. Tsukaguchi, K., de, L.B., Boom, W.H. "Differential Regulation Of IFN-Gamma, TNF-Alpha, And IL-10 Production By CD4(+) Alphabe- Tatcr+ T Cells And Vdelta2(+) Gammadelta T Cells In Response To Monocytes Infected With Mycobacterium Tuberculosis-H37Ra." Cell Immunology. 1999; 194: 12–20.

51. Wickens K, Barry D, Friezema A, et al. "Fast Foods–Are They A Risk Factor For Asthma?" Allergy. 2005; 60(12): 1537-1541.

52. Willett WC. "The Mediterranean Diet: Science And Practice." Public Health Nutrition. 2006; 9(1a): 105-110.

53. Wu, J.J., Bennett, A.M., 2005. "Essential role for mitogen-activated protein (MAP) kinase phosphatase-1 in stress-responsive MAP kinase and cell survival signaling." The Journal Biological Chemistry 280, 16461–16466.

54. Wu, L., Liu, H., Xue, P., Lu, Z.G., Du, K.F., 2001. "Influence of a triplesuperimposeded treatment on HBV replication and mutation during treating chronic hepatitis B." Zhonghua Shi Yan He Lin Chuang Bing Du Xue Za Zhi 15, 236–238.

55. Xu, F., Zhang, Y., Xiao, S., Lu, X., Yang, D., Yang, X., Li, C., Shang, M., Tu, P., Cai, S., 2006. "Absorption and metabolism of Astragali radix decoction: in silico, in vitro, and a case study in vivo." Drug Metabolism and Disposition 34, 913–924.

56. Yang, D.Z., 1993. "Effect of Astragalus membranaceuson myoelectric activity of small intestine." Zhongguo Zhong Xi Yi Jie He Za Zhi 13, 616–617.

57. Yoshida, Y., Wang, M.Q., Liu, J.N., Shan, B.E., Yamashita, U., 1997. "Immunomodulating activity of Chinese medicinal herbs and Oldenlandiadiffusain particular." International Journal of Immunopharmacology 19, 359.

58. Zhang, J.G., Yang, N., He, H., Wei, G.H., Gao, D.S., Wang, X.L., Wang, X.Z., Song, G.Y., 2005. "Effect of Astragalus injection on plasma levels of apoptosis-related factors in aged patients with chronic heart failure." Chinese Journal of Integrative Medicine 11, 187–190.

Website Resources:

1. https://www.drweil.com
2. https://www.arthritis.org/living-with-arthritis/arthritis-diet/anti-inflammatory/anti-inflammatory-diet.php
3. https://www.health.harvard.edu/staying-healthy/foods-that-fight-inflammation
4. https://www.health.com/nutrition/anti-inflammatory-diet
5. https://diet.mayoclinic.org/diet/home/google/?promo=73 3C91F8-C74E-4B52-8505-056DBE52CFA5&xid=googlesearch&awardid=google&visit _id=search&gclid=Cj0KCQiAmuHhBRD0ARIsAFWyPwg0X0 dhhSVrJu4WUsvR_YNTvj_gbayol0jKqYeBTUn0sAU7NA6YN ykaAlRvEALw_wcB
6. https://www.webmd.com/diet/anti-inflammatory-diet-road-to-good-health
7. https://www.endocrineweb.com/news/diabetes/60722-mediterranean-diet-anti-inflammatory-foods-behind-health-benefits
8. https://my.clevelandclinic.org/health/transcripts/2748_th e-anti-inflammatory-diet-a-way-to-manage-chronic-pain
9. https://www.psoriasis.org/treating-psoriasis/complementary-and-alternative/diet-and-nutrition/anti-inflammatory-diet
10. https://multiplesclerosisnewstoday.com/2017/09/06/will -you-try-an-anti-inflammatory-diet-for-your-multiple-sclerosis/
11. https://www.fammed.wisc.edu/files/webfm-uploads/documents/outreach/im/handout_ai_diet_patient. pdf
12. https://www.umassmed.edu/nutrition/ibd/ibdaid/

Contemporary Article Resources:

1. Eating Well: "The Anti-Inflammatory Diet: Is It Right for You?" http://www.eatingwell.com/article/290509/the-anti-inflammatory-diet-is-it-right-for-you/
2. Mind Body Green: "Anti-Inflammatory Diets: 11 Rules for Optimal Health" https://www.mindbodygreen.com/0-22607/antiinflammatory-diets-11-rules-for-optimal-health.html
3. Food Revolution Network: "Fight Disease with an Anti-Inflammatory Diet + 7 Foods That Fight Inflammation" https://foodrevolution.org/blog/anti-inflammatory-diet-foods-that-fight-inflammation/
4. Tufts University: "Anti-Inflammatory Diets: Do They Work?" https://www.nutritionletter.tufts.edu/issues/14_1/current-articles/Anti-Inflammatory-Diets-Do-They-Work_2286-1.html
5. Journal of the Academy of Nutrition and Dietetics: "What is the Anti-Inflammatory Diet?" https://jandonline.org/article/S0002-8223(10)01555-5/fulltext
6. Very Well Health: "The Anti-Inflammatory Diet: Can the Foods You Eat Beat Inflammation?" https://www.verywellhealth.com/anti-inflammatory-diet-88752
7. Medical News Today: "Anti-Inflammatory Diet: What to Know" https://www.medicalnewstoday.com/articles/320233.php
8. Arivale: "9 Rules for Following an Anti-Inflammatory Diet" https://www.arivale.com/blog/anti-inflammatory-diet-rules
9. The Chopra Center: "The Do's and Don't's of an Anti-Inflammatory Diet" https://chopra.com/articles/the-dos-and-donts-of-an-anti-inflammation-diet
10. High Ya: "Anti-Inflammatory Diet: A Comprehensive Beginner's Guide"https://www.highya.com/articles-

guides/anti-inflammatory-diet-a-comprehensive-beginners-guide

11. Science Daily: "Anti-Inflammatory Diet Linked to Reduced Risk of Early Death" https://www.sciencedaily.com/releases/2018/09/180913 113815.htm

12. She Knows: "The Anti-Inflammatory Diet: Eating Foods to Heal Your Body" https://www.sheknows.com/health-and-wellness/articles/803649/the-anti-inflammatory-diet-eating-foods-to-heal-your-body/

13. The Whole U, at the University of Washington: "FightinInflammationon with Food" https://www.washington.edu/wholeu/2016/09/28/fighting-inflammation-with-food/

14. Bulletproof: "Anti-Inflammatory Foods" https://blog.bulletproof.com/anti-inflammatory-foods-pain/

15. Integrative Pain Science Institute: "The Evidence supporting the Anti-Inflammatory Diet" https://www.integrativepainscienceinstitute.com/anti-inflammatory-diet-evidence/

16. The Globe and the Mail: "Anti-Inflammatory Diet May Guard Against Cancer" https://www.theglobeandmail.com/life/health-and-fitness/article-anti-inflammatory-diet-may-guard-against-cancer/

17. Science Direct: "An Anti-Inflammatory Diet as a Potential Intervention for Depressive Disorders: A Systematic Review and Meta-Analysis" https://www.sciencedirect.com/science/article/pii/S0261 561418325408

18. John Hopkins Health Review: "Understanding Inflammation" https://www.johnshopkinshealthreview.com/issues/spring-summer-2016/articles/understanding-inflammation

19. Medscape: "The Anti-Inflammatory Diet's Surprising Benefits in Children" https://www.medscape.com/viewarticle/894241
20. Root + Revel: "What is an Anti-Inflammatory Diet" https://rootandrevel.com/what-is-an-anti-inflammatory-diet/
21. Wild Earth Medicine: "Anti-Inflammatory Diet Plan: Getting Started" https://www.wildearthacupuncture.com/blog/2018/4/24/anti-inflammatory-diet-plan
22. Experience Life: "Fighting Inflammation" https://experiencelife.com/article/fighting-inflammation/
23. Arthritis Health: "An Anti-Inflammatory Diet for Arthritis" https://www.arthritis-health.com/treatment/diet-and-nutrition/anti-inflammatory-diet-arthritis
24. Garretson Food Center and Catering, Health and Wellness: "Anti-Inflammatory Q&A" https://garretsonfoodcenter.com/health_wellness/articles/273/anti-inflammatory-diet-qa
25. Today's Dietician: "Inflammation and Cancer Risk: Can Anti-Inflammatory Diets Help?" https://www.todaysdietitian.com/newarchives/0118p12.shtml
26. Lose Weight By Eating: "Top 10 Anti-Inflammatory Foods (#1 I My Favorite" https://loseweightbyeating.com/anti-inflammatory-diet-top-10-foods/
27. Active: "The Anti-Inflammatory Benefits of a Plant-based Diet" https://www.active.com/nutrition/articles/the-anti-inflammatory-benefits-of-a-plant-based-diet
28. Mosaic Science: "Eat to Treat" https://mosaicscience.com/story/eat-treat-diet-inflammation-diabetes/
29. Practical Pain Management: "An Anti-Inflammatory Diet for Pain Patients"

https://www.practicalpainmanagement.com/treatments/complementary/anti-inflammatory-diet-pain-patients

30. University Health News Daily: "Anti-Inflammatory Foods: Do They Work?" https://universityhealthnews.com/daily/nutrition/anti-inflammatory-foods/

31. Sage Journals: "Barriers and Facilitators to an Anti-Inflammatory Diet for Individuals with Spinal Cord Injuries" https://journals.sagepub.com/doi/full/10.1177/2055102918798732

32. Frontier in Psychiatry: "A Pro-Inflammatory Diet is Associated with an Increased Odds of Depression Symptoms among Iranian Female Adolescents: A Cross-sectional Study" https://www.frontiersin.org/articles/10.3389/fpsyt.2018.00400/full

33. American Society for Nutrition: "Inflammation: What is it, and How Can My Diet and Behavior Affect It?" https://nutrition.org/inflammation-what-is-it-and-how-can-my-diet-and-behavior-affect-it/

34. Weil A.: "Anti-Inflammatory Diet and Food Pyramid." http://www.drweil.com/drw/u/ART02995/Dr-Weil-Anti-Inflammatory-Food-Pyramid.html

35. Gastrointestinal Journal: "Adherence to an Anti-Inflammatory Diet Prevents Increases in Colonic Inflammation in Ulcerative Colitis Patients in Remission" https://www.gastrojournal.org/article/S0016-5085(17)32142-X/fulltext

36. Gastro Health: "Anti-Inflammatory Diet" https://gastrohealth.com/anti-inflammatory-diet-2/

37. Oxford Academic: "Following an Anti-Inflammatory Diet Prevents Increases of Fecal Calprotectin and Alters Metabolomic Profile of Ulcerative Colitis Patients, a Randomized Controlled Trial" https://academic.oup.com/jcag/article/1/suppl 2/25/4916515

38. Peak Fitness Presented by Mercola: "Exercise and Diet Combat Inflammation, Allowing You to Live Longer"https://fitness.mercola.com/sites/fitness/archive/2015/08/21/exercise-diet-inflammation.aspx

Conclusion

Thank you again for downloading this book, *The Easy Anti-Inflammatory Diet for Beginners: A No-Stress Meal Plan with Easy Recipes to Heal the Immune System!*

As you combed through the pages of this book, you have been introduced to a variety of tips and techniques for embracing the anti-inflammatory diet to make your life healthier and balanced. The unfortunate part about living in a society that encourages Western diet philosophies and lifestyle habits means that just about everyone suffers from a form of chronic inflammation. This "bad" inflammation is what is hurting and even killing your body.

Now that you know what inflammation is and how to embrace the anti-inflammatory diet, it is time to start making the changes. Your next step is to begin replacing your foods in your kitchen, following the advice in chapter 5. This simple start can help ease you into the lifestyle with foods that are going to start healing your body rather than hurting it. After you begin re-stocking your kitchen with these helpful ingredients, you will be ready to take on the two-week meal plan and diet introduction in chapter 6. As you begin adopting this way of life you will begin to notice how healthy you are feeling. And an added benefit is how great you will look, too!

Battling the chronic inflammation that has been building in your body for years is a long-term commitment. Your body has taken all this time to feed into the chronic inflammation and harm your body; it is going to take time for it to reverse the damage that has been done. Depending on your ailments, it can take months or even years to reverse harm. As you begin supporting your body rather than harming it, practice patience and kindness to yourself. You are making decisions for your long-term health and future. But the good news is that this life is full of flavor and variety! You still can have a plate full of tasty foods and enjoy eating in a whole new way.

Finally, if you enjoyed this book, then I would like to ask you for a favor; would you be kind enough to leave a review for this book on Amazon? It would be greatly appreciated!

CPSIA information can be obtained
at www.ICGtesting.com
Printed in the USA
BVHW040216201219
567307BV00016B/349/P

9 781794 468948